Carb Cycling Lifestyle for Women

A Painless Diet Plan to Lose Weight and Enjoy Your Life

John Carver

Table of Contents

INTRODUCTION 1

   ABOUT THE AUTHOR.. 4

   A FITNESS MOVEMENT FOR WOMEN 6

CHAPTER 1: WELCOME TO CARB CYCLING............................ 9

   WHAT IS CARB CYCLING AND HOW DO YOU DO IT?...................... 11

      Current Body Mass/Fat Levels.. 12

      Body Mass/Composition Goals 12

      Training Schedule 13

      Training Intensity 13

      Fitness Events/Competitions 13

   WHAT MAKES CARB CYCLING SO EFFECTIVE? 15

      The Science Behind Carb Cycling 15

   THE DIFFERENCE BETWEEN CARB CYCLING AND KETO 18

      A Deep Dive Into Ketosis.. 18

      Getting Fat From Carbs 19

      Why Ketosis is Good for Weight Loss 19

      Keto vs. Carb Cycling: Which Is better? 20

      The Middle Ground: Keto Cycling 21

   THE HIGHS AND LOWS OF CARB CYCLING 22

      High-Carb Days... 22

      Low-Carb Days 23

      Shifting Cycles 23

   IS CARB CYCLING FOR YOU? 25

      Pros of Carb Cycling... 25

      Cons of Carb Cycling.. 27

      Should You Give It a Try?... 28

   FINAL THOUGHTS 30

CHAPTER 2: TAILORING IT TO WOMEN 31

   WHY CARB CYCLING IS DIFFERENT FOR WOMEN 33

      The Protection of the Thyroid 34

Female Insulin Sensitivity 34

Getting Fit for Women 36

MASTERING THE ART OF CYCLE SYNCING 38

Benefits of Cycle Syncing..38

Foods to Avoid for Cycle Syncing 39

Finding Your Phase 40

Menstrual Phase..40

Follicular Phase...41

Ovulation Phase 42

Luteal Phase 42

FINAL THOUGHTS 44

CHAPTER 3: PRINCIPLES BEHIND PLANNING........................ 45

BREAKING THE CYCLE DOWN ACCORDING TO MACROS.....................47

What Are Macros? 47

Determining Your TDEE or Total Daily Energy Expenditure 49

Calculating Your Macros 51

Ideal Macros for High and Low Days...................................52

HOW TO MAKE A DIET PLAN...56

SAMPLE WEEKLY MEAL PLAN 59

Day 1: Low-Carb Day..59

Day 2: High-Carb Day 60

Day 3: High-Carb Day 60

Day 4: Low-Carb Day..61

Day 5: High-Carb Day 61

Day 6: High-Carb Day 62

Day 7: Low-Carb Day..62

FINAL THOUGHTS 63

AUTHOR'S NOTE 64

CHAPTER 4: CREATE YOUR OWN PLAN 64

THINGS TO REMEMBER WHEN MAKING YOUR OWN DIET PLAN 68

There Are Many Different Factors to Consider When Deciding on High
and Low Intervals 68

Carb Cycling Isn't the Same as Keto..69

Carb Cycling Is Different for Women than It Is for Men 70

It Would Be Best to Sync Carb and Menstrual Cycles.....................70

On High-Carb Days, Eat Little Fat... and Vice-Versa......................70

Don't Overcomplicate Things 71

STEP-BY-STEP GUIDE TO MAKING YOUR CARB CYCLING PLAN 72

Step 1: Know Your Vital Statistics...72

Step 2: Establish Your Goals...73

Step 3: Set Your Training Regimen 74

Step 4: Find Your Total Daily Energy Expenditure (TDEE) 74

Step 5: Find Your Total Daily Caloric Intake 75

Step 6: Calculate Your Macros for High- and Low-Carb Days 76

Step 7: Figure Out Your Menstrual Cycle Phases 77

Step 8: Plot Out Your High- and Low-Carb Days............................77

Step 9: Plan Your Meals Accordingly..78

Step 10: Review Your Plan and Make Sure Everything Is Done Right 78

BEST FOOD SOURCES FOR CARBOHYDRATES 80

Carbs to Eat 81

Carbs to Avoid 82

FINAL THOUGHTS 83

CHAPTER 5: HIGH- AND LOW-CARB RECIPES........................84

BREAKFAST...85

4-Egg and Cheese Omelette with Toast Slices (Low Carb) 85

Cream Cheese Pancakes (Low Carb) 86

Keto Coconut Porridge (Low Carb) 87

Fruity Oatmeal Bowl (High Carb) 88

LUNCH 89

Zucchini and Walnut Salad (Low Carb) 89

Salad in a Jar (Low Carb) 91

Moroccan Couscous with Flank Steak (High Carb).......................... 92

Slow-Cooked Chicken and Rice Casserole (High Carb) 94

DINNER... 96

Turkey Sandwich on Whole Wheat (Low Carb) 96

Fried Kale and Broccoli Salad (Low Carb) 98

Sweet and Spicy Beef Bowl (High Carb) 100

Spicy Avocado Chicken Salad Wrap..102

SNACKS 103

Almond Milkshake (Low Carb) 103

Low-Carb Deviled Eggs (Low Carb) 104

Peanut Butter Sandwich on Wheat Bread (High Carb) 105

Multigrain Bread with Olive Oil..106

CHAPTER 6: TIPS AND TRICKS FOR SUCCESS 107

Drink Lots of Water 107

Set Concrete and Realistic Goals...108

Don't Pay Too Much Attention to the Scale....................................108

Do Meal Planning and Preparation...109

Remember Fat Isn't the Enemy...110

Stick to a Solid Workout Plan..111

Cook Your Own Meals 111

Avoid Drinking Calories 112

Don't Go Grocery Shopping While Hungry or Without a Plan........113

Evolve Your Goals Along the Way 113

Don't Give Up on a Diet Too Quickly 114

Find Yourself a Diet or Training Buddy..115

Stick to Workouts or Diets You Really Enjoy 115

Schedule Your Cheat Days...116

Get Better Sleep at Night..117

FINAL THOUGHTS...118

AUTHOR'S NOTE 119

CONCLUSION 120

REFERENCES 123

Introduction

Weight loss might still be an incredibly sensitive and taboo topic for a lot of people. These days, you have to be very careful when you talk about a person's weight because you never know when you might offend someone. However, in spite of that, more and more people are starting to adopt healthier lifestyles and are more open to discussing the harsh realities of getting fit and healthy. Because the truth is that while we picture fit and healthy people as always so happy and positive, the road to getting fit is not a glamorous one. It's harsh. It's a struggle. And unfortunately, this is the reason why a lot of people just end up quitting a short time after they begin. They realize that their expectations were false to begin with, and they become disappointed when their results are not up to par.

This book is going to help you manage your expectations better so that you not only go into your weight loss journey with the right approach, but you also go into it with the right mindset. Remember that mindset makes up a huge part of the game. You need to have the proper disposition going into any difficult endeavor if you are hoping to find success in it. Of course, more than just telling you what to do to be healthier, this book is also going to orient you on the many things that you need to prepare your mind for to tackle this problem. And make no mistake about it, obesity really is a problem.

People shouldn't have to be shamed by others for wanting to lose weight. It's the same as when someone enrolls in school to learn about a new academic field or when someone takes up a new hobby to master a new craft. People who go on diets or undergo physical exercise regimens are just people who are seeking to make their lives better. They understand that there is a problem with the way that they are living their lives and that there is room for improvement. And don't doubt the fact that so many people in the world have problems with their weight.

According to data that was published in *The Lancet* journal, more than 3.4 million human deaths worldwide were caused by overweight- or obesity-related diseases in 2014 (Afshin et al., 2019). The same data set that was published in the article revealed that there have been 27.5% and 47.1% upticks in the number of overweight and obese adults and children respectively since 1980. Those are alarming numbers and the statistics don't make for very good future prospects in health and fitness. Obesity is a very serious public health issue that needs to be addressed on both a policy level and a personal level. According to the World Obesity Federation, more than $850 billion is spent per year on direct healthcare costs for people who are obese or overweight (World Economic Forum, 2018). So, obesity isn't just a matter of compromising one's physical health. It's also compromising peoples' financial well-being as well.

However, as echoed in an article published by the World Economic Forum, the common sentiment is not that people don't have the willpower or the conviction to want to be healthy (Ryan, Candeias, & Jorgensen, 2018). A lot of the blame regarding why obesity persists in being a global problem today rests on the fact that there are still a lot of misinformation and outdated perceptions on health and wellness. All of these conflicting data and ideas have accounted for people to lead very unhealthy lives even though they believe they are doing the opposite. This is why there is a need to further push for more science-backed recommendations on how to tackle weight loss and obesity. Hence, this book.

Of course, there are a myriad of literary sources out there that are available for your consumption. Why should you trust this one in particular? We've already talked about how in this age of information, there are certain dangers surrounding misinformation and the peddling of fake news. Naturally, you should be skeptical of everything that you read, right? That's only natural. No one would blame you for wanting to authenticate everything that you read, especially when it concerns your health and well-being.

So, in an attempt to assuage your apprehensions and skepticism, perhaps it would be a good idea for you to get to know the person behind the words that you're currently reading.

About the Author

John Carver is a health expert and author who was born and raised on the island of Bermuda. He completed his tertiary studies at university in Washington, DC, and took his professional practice to California where he got a job for a prominent retail company. It was during this early stage of his career wherein he really dedicated himself to the realms of health and fitness. He embarked on a very vigorous training and exercise program as he set bigger and higher goals for himself.

However, it was only after a friend had given him insights into how his diet was affecting his physical performance during training when John quickly realized that his approach was lacking in something vital. He discovered that he also needed to be paying just as much attention to the food that he was eating as well. It wasn't just about the effort that he was putting into his training sessions. It was also about the fuel and the nutrients that he was putting into his body. This is when John decided that he needed to change his outlook and take a new approach to his fitness.

A new enterprise—selling health supplements—along with an enhanced training regimen, meant that John took much greater care of what he ate and in particular of the carbohydrates he consumed. That, in turn, led to much better performances in the competitions he entered, but the biggest change came when he decided to spread his knowledge and share his experiences to a wider audience.

His book, *Carb Cycling: The Science and Practice of Mastering Your Metabolism*, has proven to be an exciting addition to books that not only help athletes look after their bodies, but also provide help for people who are keen to lose weight and take care of themselves better. Of course, the dietary needs of different people are going to differ based on the kinds of lives that they lead. This is a point that John has stressed in depth in his books. However, through his guidance and education, plenty of people, regardless of fitness backgrounds or athletic levels, have managed to find success in their own personal fitness goals.

Given the impact that he has made on countless lives, John is planning other books along the same lines and is embarking on expanding his business further. He hopes that by doing so, he will reach out to even more people who will reap the same rewards that he has.

In his spare time, John enjoys running, cooking, and spending lots of time with his girlfriend. He loves nothing better than spending days at the beach, grilling food on an open fire, and watching the stars with an occasional cold beer and great friends around him.

A Fitness Movement for Women

Again, it's important to emphasize the fact that different people are going to have different needs and prescriptions when it comes to their fitness activities or dietary practices. This is why this book isn't going to be in the business of providing any cookie-cutter advice that is aimed at a general audience. The information and advice that will be listed here should be fit for women, in particular, who are looking to get healthier and fitter through carb cycling.

When it comes to health and wellness, one must always consider the fact that certain practices are only effective depending on the physiological responses of the human body. And given that men and women have very different physical makeups, it's important to emphasize that the approaches to health and fitness for each gender are more specialized and streamlined relative to the ways that their bodies are constructed. This book goes the extra mile by providing some very key insights into how women's bodies are constructed and how they adapt to certain fitness and dietary programs. You must realize that achieving health and wellness is a very nuanced endeavor and that there are many nuances to dieting and exercising. It can be very overwhelming to have to gather, absorb, and practice all of these nuances that come from scattered sources. This is why this book is going to curate all of the information and knowledge that you need to know in order for you to really find success in your health and wellness goals.

The road to achieving optimal health and wellness is not an easy one. And it definitely isn't one that guarantees immediate success either. It's a lot of ups and downs, rises and falls, highs and lows. Sure, you might find success in the initial phases of it, but you shouldn't expect your success to be consistent or linear. Expect a lot of speed bumps, setbacks, and major hurdles in this journey of yours. However, you shouldn't fret. It's important that you understand the value of embracing the process. As early as now, you need to develop the conviction that is necessary to carry you through the tough journey that you're going to take. It's definitely not going to be without its fair share of difficulties. But nothing worth having in life ever comes easily anyway.

You shouldn't let the difficulty or enormity of the challenge that faces you be intimidating enough to make you want to give up. This is why this book and many others like it exist. This book is going to guide you through every step of the way. Remember that whenever you are faced with a wall that you feel like you can't overcome, someone else has stood exactly where you are right now. And that same person has managed to overcome that wall to keep on pushing through. If it can work for them, then it should also work for you.

Carb cycling is a scientifically proven and trusted method for losing weight and getting healthier. Not only that, it has also managed to help athletes all over the world improve their athletic performance significantly. These improvements have led them to break through walls and barriers that were previously impervious to their efforts. Sure, you can always lose a few pounds here and there by exercising really hard and committing to a strict training regimen. But if you don't have a diet that is able to properly nourish you and supplement your workouts, then you won't really be able to maximize your potential.

So, this is why one must always need to take a holistic and well-rounded approach to getting fit. You can't be a great exerciser without paying attention to the food that you eat. And you can't be a healthy eater if you're just going to end up not using any of your calories and sitting around all day. Diet and exercise are two things that go hand-in-hand. And there are all sorts of diet and exercise programs out there that many people have found success in. However, for the woman who is looking for an effective and sustainable way of achieving all her health and wellness goals, there is carb cycling. If you are ready to take a deep dive into the world of carb cycling, then let's journey into the first chapter of this book together.

Chapter 1:
Welcome to Carb Cycling

If you're a parent, you would never allow your small child to dive into a pool without knowing how deep it is first, right? When you're sick, you never want to take any medicine without first understanding how it's going to affect your body. When you see a nice pair of expensive shoes at a designer store that you're interested in, you want to find out everything you need to know about that shoe before you pour a lot of money into buying it. This is the same kind of approach that anyone should take to adopting a new diet or exercise routine. You don't want to dive into carb cycling without first understanding the principles behind it. You should always orient and familiarize yourself first with all that there is to know about carb cycling so that you are tackling and approaching it the right way.

Of course, it's not just about ensuring your own safety and wellness. Sure, there are certain diets out there that might prove to be effective for certain types of people but can be just as dangerous for others. For example, a high-protein or high-fat diet might not exactly be ideal for a patient with kidney disease even though these tend to be very popular "weight loss" diets for most other people. A Mediterranean diet, which is high in carbs, isn't going to be the best one for patients who are diabetic or who have high blood sugar levels. However, there are plenty of others who will swear that adopting the Mediterranean diet has helped them become fitter and healthier. Again, it all depends on the person and how their body responds to a certain diet.

Prior to trying out carb cycling, you first have to determine if it's the right diet for you. And the first step to doing so is making sure that you understand all of the key information and details surrounding carb cycling. From there, you will have a more refined and insightful opinion on the matter.

However, more than just knowing if it would be a safe and plausible diet for you, it's important that you approach the diet the right way. You will never be able to find success in any endeavor if you don't take the time to properly familiarize and orient yourself with it first. There are plenty of novices out there who only read the headlines surrounding certain diet fads without acquainting themselves with the fine print. They end up approaching the diet the wrong way, and they don't get the results that were promised to them. You never want to fall into the same kind of trap. A huge part of finding success in a difficult endeavor such as this is making sure that you have all bases covered with regards to your approach to it.

This is exactly what this chapter is going to try to help you out with. If you're coming from a place where you know absolutely nothing about carb cycling, then there's no need to worry. By the time you finish reading this chapter, you will be in a much better position than before. You will be briefed on the idea of carb cycling and how it impacts your body to help stimulate weight loss and improved athletic performance. You will also be exposed to the science behind carb cycling and why it works for so many people. Don't worry. You don't need a degree in nutrition or biomechanics to understand the science behind it. This chapter is also going to delve deeper into the effectiveness of carb cycling relative to other similar diet styles.

All of this information is valuable knowledge that will allow you to determine whether this is the diet for you. This knowledge is also going to help you on your path should you proceed to go this route towards health and fitness. Now, this prompts us to ask the question, what exactly is carb cycling?

What Is Carb Cycling and How Do You Do It?

Carbs have been demonized by the health and fitness community for the longest time now. You probably hear about it all the time. *Lay off the carbs. Cut out the sugar. Stop eating donuts.* Carbs have really gotten a bad rep in the dieting world. But is all that hate really warranted? There are all sorts of popular diet programs out there that dramatically restrict carbohydrate consumption. Heck, there are even certain diets out there that get rid of carbs altogether. Are carbs really all that bad?

Just in case you don't already know, carbs actually comprise just one of the three macronutrients that should be making up your daily diet. The other macronutrients are proteins and fats. Given that, it's important to emphasize that there is no one macronutrient that is inherently unhealthy or bad. All macronutrients, or *macros,* have their place in the nourishment of the human body. These macros all serve very distinct and specific purposes. It's only when humans overindulge or abuse the consumption of certain macros that it becomes bad and unhealthy.

Essentially, the carb cycling diet program is based on the principle that carbohydrates don't necessarily have to be restricted per se. The consumption of carbs under carb cycling just has to be managed and tailored properly relative to the needs of the individual. To be more concrete about it, people who go through carb cycling just alternate the intervals wherein they maximize and minimize their carb consumptions.

The durations of these intervals can vary depending on the individual. Some people cycle through their carbs on a daily, weekly, biweekly, or even monthly basis. Ultimately, the whole point of carb cycling is to stimulate fat burn while also improving athletic performance in spite of caloric restrictions. At the same time, carb cycling is a sustainable means of tackling weight loss plateaus. Typically, people who go on diets and don't change things up after sustained success are bound to hit a weight loss plateau. Essentially, a plateau takes place whenever the body adapts or acclimates itself to the dietary habits of an individual to the point where it starts burning less fat in an effort to retain more fat reserves. This is just the body's natural response to make sure that there is a lot of stored energy left in the body in case of emergencies. Of course, if you are looking to sustain weight loss for the long term, you need to break through these plateaus. And this is where carb cycling can be very effective.

Again, keep in mind that carbohydrates are not inherently bad. All macros serve a very distinct and specific purpose. However, what the carb cycling method does is minimize one's chances of consuming carbohydrates in excess and during times when they don't really need it. Through a popular carb cycling program, one would only consume carbohydrates during moments when they provide maximum benefits and in the proper degrees. There are a variety of factors that can influence the manner in which you might structure your carb cycling program. Here are just some of them:

Current Body Mass/Fat Levels

For the casual person who is trying to lose weight, they only need to look at the current state of their bodies. Again, it's going to differ depending on how your body is currently structured. However, the general rule of thumb here is that the leaner you are, then the higher number of high-carb consumption intervals or blocks you would have.

Body Mass/Composition Goals

This is a variable that factors in greatly to those who are really looking to chisel their physiques to the greatest level of detail. This carb cycling variable is most important to bodybuilders who are training for competitions or events. Essentially, they divide their carb cycling into phases depending on where they are in their training regimen. For mass bulking and bodybuilding, one would increase carb consumption. And for mass cutting, one would minimize carb consumption as much as possible.

Training Schedule

Another big factor that most people consider when plotting out their carb cycling intervals is the training schedule. One general principle that people follow is that they maximize carb consumption on training days, and they minimize carb consumption on rest days. The principle behind this is that the body doesn't need as many carbohydrates to function and perform properly when it isn't put through a strenuous workout. So, it would be best to minimize carb consumption during these days.

Training Intensity

Sometimes, it's not just a matter of consuming large amounts of carbohydrates on training days and restricting carbs on rest days. Some athletes will really go into detail by factoring in the level of intensity that they exert during workouts on certain days. However, the principles of carb cycling still remain consistent. The more intense or more physically demanding a training session is, then the higher the demand for carbohydrates on that day. Conversely, when training sessions are light and relatively easy, then the lower the requirements for carbs.

Fitness Events/Competitions

This variable of carb cycling might be just for a select group of people but it's still worth mentioning. There are certain athletes out there who just aren't training to be fit or healthy. There are athletes who are training towards competitions or sporting events. Sometimes, they will structure their carb cycling patterns based on the schedule of their competitions and events. Some athletes might overindulge on carbs in the lead-up to endurance-based events like marathons or triathlons. Some athletes might cut out carbs in the lead-up to certain events like bodybuilding competitions or photo shoots.

What Makes Carb Cycling So Effective?

Sure, now you may get the basic gist of what carb cycling is and how people incorporate it into their daily lives. Now, we ask the question: how does it work? Earlier, we discussed how carb cycling is a dietary pattern that is proven to be effective for many different people who have differing goals. If you're someone who is trying to train for an athletic competition, carb cycling can help fuel your athletic performance. If you're someone who has to lose some weight quickly for a special event, carb cycling can help you get the job done. Even if you're just someone who wants to stay trim and healthy over a sustainable period, carb cycling can help you out with that as well.

It seems too good to be true that a simple carb consumption pattern can impact so many kinds of people with different goals in a positive manner. However, it shouldn't be too difficult to believe in the carb cycling philosophy once you take the time to understand the science behind it and how it affects your body.

The Science Behind Carb Cycling

Compared to other mainstream dietary programs and philosophies, carb cycling is relatively new. This means that the scientific data surrounding carb cycling may not be as exhaustive as compared to those of diets like keto or Paleo. However, as you continue to read on, you will learn that the evidence is actually compelling enough to make a solid case for itself in terms of effectiveness and sustainability. Essentially, all of the scientific principles surrounding carb cycling have to do with the natural bodily reactions that are associated with the manipulation of carbohydrate consumption.

Before you can understand the science behind carb cycling, you must first understand what carbs are and why the body needs them in the first place. Essentially, in order for your body to function properly, it needs energy. Your body gets this energy from glucose. The glucose that your body converts into energy comes from the calories that you consume on a daily basis. Your calories stem mostly from your macronutrients that we have already discussed earlier: protein, fat, and carbohydrates. However, the macronutrient that has the most efficient properties for glucose conversion is carbs. So, this is why a lot of people tend to associate carbohydrates with energy. When the body is deprived of calories to convert into glucose, it targets the reserves (the body's accumulated fats) and converts those into glucose for energy instead.

So, with that in mind, this is where carb cycling comes in. Ideally, when plotting a carb cycling program, one would manipulate carb consumption levels relative to the demands of the body. When the body doesn't need too much energy to perform or function adequately, then carb consumption must be managed to meet those needs and not exceed them. The reason that carbs should ideally be limited on nonintense days (or rest days) is because the body doesn't really need to expend much energy to function properly. Hence, any excess carbohydrates or glucose might end up getting converted to stored fat instead. This could be problematic for anyone whose goals are to get leaner and trimmer, especially around the waist.

However, it's not just about losing weight. Again, athletes who care about their physical performance may also engage in carb cycling. This is where high-carb days during the carb cycling program come in. Usually, when workouts get really strenuous, athletes will struggle with recovery and rejuvenation to sustain a long-term training plan. Consuming large amounts of carbohydrates can aid in refueling the glycogen in muscles. This means that muscles aren't broken down so much and are quicker at recovering for more workouts.

There is also another layer to the carb cycling method, and it has something to do with hormone manipulation in the body. Leptin and ghrelin are hormones that regulate a person's weight and appetite and that are produced within the body. Through strategic carb cycling, the production of these hormones is regulated optimally so as to stimulate fat burn while also suppressing unnecessary hunger pangs.

During low-carb days, the body is sometimes forced to enter a carb-fasted state. At its most extreme form, this is sometimes referred to as ketosis wherein the body's liver produces ketones which serve as the replacements for glucose that comes from carbohydrates. In order to produce ketones, the body has to burn off stored fat in the body. This is where fat loss is at its most optimal. Instead of relying on the calories that one consumes for energy, the body tries to become more self-sustaining by burning off more of its reserves instead. However, low-carb consumption days on a carb cycling diet don't really call for one to enter a state of ketosis. Those are only requirements of a keto diet. But more on that later. Ultimately, it is said that carb cycling can help stimulate the body's metabolism and burn fat at a more efficient rate.

Lastly, the final scientific layer to the effectiveness of carb cycling has to do with insulin sensitivity. Essentially, by strategically minimizing or cutting out carbs from a diet, the body's insulin levels are regulated properly so as not to induce weight gain, diabetes, or heart disease.

The Difference Between Carb Cycling and Keto

If you've already done your research about dieting and fitness prior to reading this book, then there is a very good chance that you've already encountered the idea of keto. It was already previously mentioned in this chapter that keto is a dietary form of restricting one's self from consuming carbohydrates so as to induce a state of ketosis in the body (or a ketogenic state). So, if keto is also a diet that promotes the minimal consumption of carbohydrates, then what makes it less or more effective than carb cycling? If carb cycling is the restriction of carb intake through intervals, wouldn't a stagnant state of restriction result in better outcomes for weight loss? These are some very valid questions, and it's definitely okay for you to be asking them. But before we get to the root of the answer, we need to dig deeper beyond the surface levels of each dietary proposition.

A Deep Dive Into Ketosis

Think of your body as a machine that runs on fuel. This fuel can come in many different forms through the food that you eat. However, your body as a machine has a natural personal preference in where it sources its fuel. For the most part, it chooses to process carbs over the other two macronutrients. The reason for that is because carbs are the easiest for the body to process into glucose, which is used to energize your body and keep the machine running operationally.

So, as has already been explained earlier, the carbs that you eat get processed into its simplest form, called glucose. This glucose is then picked up and pushed through your bloodstream to distribute energy all throughout your body. However, not all of this glucose is used up by your body, especially on days when you're not being physically active. This is when your glucose ends up getting stored as fat.

Getting Fat From Carbs

Once your body has determined that all of your caloric needs are met, whatever glucose is left behind doesn't get used up and is stored in the body's reserves. So, if we go back to the analogy of the machine, when you're taking in too much glucose, you are going to start overflowing with fuel. All of that excess energy has to go somewhere. Naturally, what the body does is it converts all of that unused glucose into stored energy called glycogen.

Later on, when your body starts running out of energy, it takes whatever stored glycogen is left and converts it back into glucose to fuel the body. Over time, if the glycogen really doesn't get used up, it turns into the visible fat that you see on your arms, waist, legs, and the rest of your body. This is why you end up getting those love handles whenever you aren't burning off more than you're eating.

Why Ketosis is Good for Weight Loss

So, given all of that information surrounding the processing of carbohydrates, simple logic will tell you that the key to losing weight would be to make sure that you're burning off more energy than you're eating. However, what ketosis does is take the fat-burning process a step further by forcing the body to burn its own reserved fats instead of the energy that you're eating through your food. Again, as has been previously mentioned, this fat-burning process by carb restriction is called putting your body into a ketogenic state.

The way that the keto diet works is that it always pushes for your body to be in a perpetual state of ketosis. This way, your body is constantly trying to burn off its reserved fats in order to sustain itself. Originally, ketosis was actually an experiment that was used to treat patients who were experiencing seizures or epilepsy. There was evidence that suggested that ketogenic patients had better experiences when dealing with seizures. However, it has mostly evolved to become a weight loss tool, especially in this modern age.

Keto vs. Carb Cycling: Which Is better?

So, to sum it all up, keto is essentially the perpetual restriction or minimization of carbohydrate consumption to induce a constant state of ketosis in the body to stimulate one's metabolism. This is why a lot of people tend to adopt the keto diet whenever they're trying to meet specific weight loss goals such as reaching a target weight on the scale or being able to fit into an old pair of jeans.

On the other hand, there is carb cycling. This is a dietary philosophy that encourages intervals of high-carb and low-carb consumption days. If you take away the component of intervals in carb cycling, it should share a lot of the same principles as the keto diet. However, there is a substantial difference in terms of execution and results. As you are plotting your carb cycling routine, you would never really aim to induce a state of ketosis in your body, not even on your low-carb days. Ketosis is not a requirement for traditional carb cycling. Also, the main difference between keto and carb cycling is the duration of carb restriction. With keto, it's a perpetual state of restriction. With carb cycling, the durations for restriction are strategically timed.

Now, it's time for us to answer the question: which one is better?

You might hate this answer, but the truth is that it depends. It really depends on the kind of goals that you have and what kind of personality you have as well. At the end of the day, it's all about being able to find a diet that works for you. Sustainability is key here. Sure, you might find immediate success with a keto diet, but would you really be able to sustain carb restrictions for the long term? Of course, you might find comfort in the carb cycling diet, but will it be able to provide you with the results that you want in the time that you set for yourself? It's all relative. Again, it all boils down to whatever works best for you. And while that may be the safe and unsatisfying answer, it's also what is true.

The Middle Ground: Keto Cycling

For those who want to marry both dieting principles, there is also such a thing as keto cycling. And it's exactly what it sounds like. Essentially, you would induce a state of ketosis in your body, but you would only do so in intervals. So, like the carb cycling scheduling format, you would have keto days and nonketo days. For a lot of people who want to reap the dramatic benefits of ketosis, this is a more sustainable way of going about it as it doesn't completely eliminate carbohydrate consumption altogether.

However, that isn't the only variable that you want to take into consideration when deciding for yourself what dietary program to undertake. There are certain pros and cons that are attached to each dietary principle which will make them more distinct. It would be best for you to gather more information about keto, carb cycling, keto cycling, and any other dietary program before you come to a decision. Again, knowledge is power.

The Highs and Lows of Carb Cycling

Ultimately, getting into a carb cycling diet just means having high carb and low carb days. The key is in making sure that all of the numbers add up and that you're distributing your high- and low-carb days properly. Again, there are a variety of factors that you need to consider when determining when your high- and low-carb days are going to be. You have to consider your current body mass composition, target body composition, training schedule, training intensity, etc. However, the general idea here is that you don't go too many consecutive days of just having either high- or low-carb consumption. You want to mix it up as much as possible.

High-Carb Days

Again, the numbers can vary from person to person. However, if you're just starting out, you won't want to stray too far away from the recommended number of 60% of calories consumed from carbohydrates. So, if you're eating 2,000 calories a day, that means you should be eating 1,200 calories from carbohydrates during high-carb days. As you gain more experience and practice in carb cycling, you can tweak the numbers to meet your specific needs as you go.

It's also important to really listen to your body when you're engaged in a strict training regimen. If you feel like you're feeling gassed just 5 minutes into a workout, it might be due to you not having enough carbs to work with. Sometimes, not having enough carbs can also translate to you feeling groggy or tired when you're at the office, and you're unable to focus on your work.

However, it's very important that you don't have a "treat yourself" mindset when determining your high-carb consumption numbers. It's very dangerous to think "I ran an extra mile today, so I get to have an extra 50g of carbs." If you have a plan, try to stick to it as much as possible. You shouldn't be in the business of rewarding yourself with food. You should merely see the food that you eat as a source of nourishment for your body. It shouldn't be a prize that you get for being disciplined. Otherwise, you would be defeating the purpose of going on a diet.

Low-Carb Days

Typically, you would want to schedule your low-carb days on those days where you aren't really expending too much energy. So, perhaps on days when you're just doing less intense exercises like light jogging, yoga, or even when you're just taking a rest from working out altogether, it would be best for you to not overindulge in carbs. So, during high-carb days, you would typically load up on complex carbohydrates that come from wheats, starches, and other similar sources. On low-carb days, you will want to exchange those complex carbs for some leafy greens, lean meats, and healthy fats like oils or nuts.

To be more concrete about it, take this as an example. During high-carb days, you might have a turkey burger on a whole-wheat bun for dinner. This would be fine on a high-carb day. However, on a low-carb day, you can take this same meal and replace the whole-wheat bun with lettuce, tomatoes, onions, low-carb dressing, and even cheese.

Shifting Cycles

One of the best parts about going on a carb cycling program is that your body has a difficult time acclimating itself to what you're doing. A lot of the time, when people just completely restrict themselves from eating for prolonged periods, their bodies adapt and try to preserve more fat instead of burning it off. So, the dieting process becomes counterproductive. But with a carb cycling program, the body rarely gets a chance to acclimate itself to the constantly changing numbers in carb consumption.

However, with that said, it's still important that you shift your cycle up every once in a while. Weight plateaus are very real, and they can still happen while you're on a carb cycling program. Keep in mind that it's a lot easier for a larger person than a smaller person to burn a certain number of calories. This is because a larger body requires more calories in order to sustain itself. So, over time, as you're losing more and more weight, your caloric needs change as well. With that, you have to adjust to your changing body too. When you notice that your carb cycling program isn't as effective as it used to be, it's time for you to shift the cycles and alter the numbers. This is the only way you're going to be able to break through the plateaus you will inevitably face.

Is Carb Cycling for You?

Now, you've already been exposed to the different principles behind carb cycling and the science behind it. However, it's normal if you're not entirely sold on carb cycling just yet. It would be irresponsible for you to just automatically buy into this concept without first taking the time to really understand the nuances involved in this diet program. This is especially true considering that there are loads of other diet programs out there that you can incorporate into your daily life. Perhaps, these diets might be better for you. That's not a problem. Again, it's all about finding something that works best for you.

Given that, there is still a lot for you to learn and discover about carb cycling in relation to whether or not it would be good for you. To help you make a decision on it, you might want to consider the pros and cons that are involved in carb cycling. Of course, when you put a particular dietary philosophy up against others, certain diets are going to have their own respective strengths and weaknesses. While carb cycling has indeed proven itself to be effective to a critical mass of people, there are still certain trade-offs when you compare it to other effective diet programs.

Pros of Carb Cycling

The first advantage of carb cycling is that it's very accessible and easy to grasp for a lot of people. Also, it's not as strict as most other mainstream diets, so it won't really intimidate a lot of people who aren't too fond of drastic lifestyle changes. Since there are still days that allot for high carb consumption, it won't really be too difficult for most people to get into.

The second pro of carb cycling is that it's very flexible. There isn't really a very strict and specific program that everyone has to follow. The key to making the carb cycling diet work for you is making sure that it is tailored to your lifestyle. So, if you have a very busy day due to your job, then that means that you don't really have the time to work out. On days like those, you can still be on a diet by designating it as a low-carb day.

Another big advantage of carb cycling is that it is able to provide the body with a metabolic system that is more optimized for weight loss and fat burn. To put it simply, losing weight is just a matter of cutting calories to make sure that you're using up more energy that you're eating. However, sustainable weight loss is a lot more complicated than that. Eventually, your body adapts to your eating habits. So, if you're minimizing your calories, your body is eventually going to catch on to what you're doing. As a result, it will slow down its metabolic rate, and that won't be good for your weight loss. However, through carb cycling, your body never gets a chance to acclimate itself to what you're doing. So, it never slows down its metabolic rate, and your weight loss is never compromised. You're not on continuous deprivation of carbohydrates when you do carb cycling. As a result, your body never really feels like it has to restrict metabolic output to maintain energy reserves.

One added pro of carb cycling is that it has proven to improve athletic performance. This might be a very appealing benefit to all the readers out there who are competitive athletes who really take their training and athletic performance seriously. One common struggle that most athletes face is trying to lose weight without compromising athletic performance. A lot of the time, when training sessions get more and more intense, athletes will have to nourish their bodies with copious amounts of food, especially carbohydrates. However, carbs are also known to lead to blood sugar spikes, and this can compromise one's weight loss goals. This is why carb cycling is so effective. It still supplies the athlete with a steady influx of carbohydrates as sustenance for their intense training. But the low-carb days act as counterweights to the high-carb days, so as to prevent weight gain and even stimulate weight loss.

Lastly, you won't really have to stop yourself from eating all of your favorite food. If you're craving a generous bowl of ice cream, then you can have some. Just make sure that you fit your ice cream into your high-carb day. Cutting out carbs in traditional diets can get really boring or limiting in the long run. Fortunately, with carb cycling, you are constantly mixing things up. So, you don't have too many restrictions that limit your options.

Cons of Carb Cycling

One of the biggest cons of carb cycling is actually a con for many other diets as well. It requires great discipline. You have to pay so much attention to planning your meals and making sure that your macro intake meets specific numbers. This might not necessarily be the best diet plan for people who are unwilling to put a lot of work and effort into the planning and preparation phase. The planning and preparation process for carb cycling diets can get really comprehensive. With most diets, people are generally eating the same amount of food every day of the week. But with carb cycling, the numbers can change from day to day. So, this means that meal plans under a carb cycling method will require another added layer of detail that you need to take into consideration. With traditional meal planning, something that you would have for lunch on Monday can also be something that you can have for lunch once or twice more throughout the week. However, with carb cycling, that might not be viable as the nutritional demands might be different.

Another con of carb cycling is the fatigue that comes with low-carb days. Certain people just aren't capable of functioning properly when they don't get their fill of carbs. This might be a problem for people who need to be on top of their game but need to stay strict with their low carb consumption on those days.

Lastly, you might not be getting some valuable nutrients that you would typically get from your carbs. Fruits are a big no-no during low-carb days. However, fruits are also great sources of vitamins and minerals that make you healthier. Given that, you might have to resort to more expensive low-carb nutritional supplements to make sure that you're still getting your fill of vitamins and minerals.

Should You Give It a Try?

To be completely blunt, carb cycling used to exclusively be used by serious athletes and bodybuilders. However, it has managed to amass a mainstream popularity and is being used even by people who only engage in exercise as a form of recreation. Again, there really is no *best* diet out there. There is only a diet that works best for you. So, is carb cycling the best one you can adopt for your own lifestyle? Well, in order to come to an answer to that question, there are a few things that you need to take into consideration.

First of all, you need to look at the overall state of your health. Carb cycling might not necessarily be the healthiest option for people who are dealing with specific physical conditions. For instance, people who have issues with their blood sugar, such as diabetes or hypoglycemia, should definitely consult with their physician before taking on a diet like this. Remember that engaging in a dramatic carb-cutting diet can really alter the blood sugar spikes of your body, and this might be dangerous to you if you have a blood-related physical condition.

In addition to that, it might not be a good idea for you to engage in this diet program if you're currently engaged in another dietary program.

For example, you might be doing intermittent fasting and you're finding success in it. So, you don't want to give up intermittent fasting, but you also want to try carb cycling. Combining dietary philosophies like these might not necessarily be the healthiest thing for you or your body.

Final Thoughts

So, that's just a general overview of what carb cycling is. Of course, this was just a very brief run through of carb cycling. If you're really looking to try it out for yourself, you need to read more about it in this book. Ideally, by now, you will have come to a more educated opinion on whether this would be a great diet for you to try out. However, the best advice that you can get on this would be to just try it out. You really have nothing to lose so long as you know that your body will be able to handle it in a healthy manner. If it turns out that you don't like the diet or it doesn't really work for you, then you can always just abandon it and try something else. However, there is a lot of upside if you find out that it really does work for you and is effective. At the end of the day, embracing fitness and health is a journey. It's an exploration. It's continuous learning and self-discovery. And as the cliché goes, if you never try, then you'll never know.

Chapter 2:
Tailoring It to Women

Again, this isn't going to be just another cookie-cutter diet book that's going to assume that all of its readers are the same and are going to reap similar results. With dieting, it's very complex. What works for one isn't necessarily going to work the same way for another. In this sense, it's very important to streamline audiences. It's important to taper the prescription according to the needs of a patient. And in this case, the audience is women.

First of all, it's important to stress that this book is not being written because women are unfit to do the same things that men are capable of doing. That's not the message that is being sent out here. Of course, women always have the capacity to match and even surpass men in terms of ability and achievement. However, it would be foolish to assume that there are no biological differences between men and women. At its core, the whole idea of genders is founded on the fact that men and women have different physical makeups. To put it simply, men and women are wired differently when it comes to their physiques. So, as a result, men and women don't necessarily undergo the same bodily processes. This means that dietary programs like carb cycling aren't going to show pure consistency from person to person.

What this chapter is going to try to do is to shed more light on why carb cycling is different for women and why the approach has to be different as well. Again, when it comes to health and wellness, there are a lot of little details that need to be tended to. You might think that carb cycling would be a principle that would provide consistent results regardless of gender. But that isn't the case. Again, there are just too many variables that impact the effectiveness of a diet. One of those variables is gender. This is especially true if your ultimate goal is weight loss. Keep in mind that hormones play a very big role when it comes to metabolism and weight loss. It's also known that women undergo more hormonal changes and fluctuations than men do. That's just one aspect of why gender plays a big role in determining the effectiveness of the diet.

Ultimately, the goal of this chapter isn't to create division or any kind of discrimination. Rather, it's to take a more nuanced approach to talking about this diet. Again, when it comes to dietary programs like these, the devil is in the details. In order for you to properly execute this diet, then you need a more comprehensive overview of the gender-centric nuances that exist.

Why Carb Cycling Is Different for Women

We've already established how carb cycling is essentially just the science of inducing weight loss through alternating high- and low-carb days. Through these alternating intervals, the human body is more optimized to metabolize food and induce proper caloric processing. When you are consistently exposing your system to low-carb days, your body has better insulin sensitivity. This will help you burn fat over a more sustainable period as your metabolic system becomes more streamlined.

However, it's very important to stress that carbs are not the enemy. In fact, there are so many women out there who need carbohydrates for their bodies to function properly. And it's absolutely essential that we stress that fact. Here are some benefits of carbohydrate consumption for women, to name a few:

- Carbs help regulate hormonal systems in women.
- Carbs aid in the recovery from hypothalamic amenorrhea.
- Carbs help alleviate complications from thyroid issues.
- Carbs are essential for healthy pregnancies, etc.

So, while carbs may contribute to weight gain to a certain degree, just eliminating them altogether wouldn't necessarily be the smartest thing to do in most cases. Given that, carb cycling offers a perceivably safe middle ground. You're not eliminating carbs from your diet, but you're meticulously controlling your consumption so as to not interfere with your desires to lose weight.

However, there is a very common mistake that most women make when they try to get into carb cycling. They don't take their gender into consideration when doing so. This is understandable. When you take a look at the fitness industry, it has a tendency to be a very male-dominated community, especially when it comes to carb cycling. This is because, as we mentioned, carb cycling originated as a dieting technique for bodybuilders and high-profile athletes. As you may already know, those fields tend to have larger male communities. So, as this diet emerged into the mainstream, more women started adopting the carb cycling diet for themselves not knowing that they needed to factor their gender into the equation.

If you are a woman who is just trying to get into carb cycling for the first time and you don't really have a female resource person to help you out with things, don't fret. This segment of the book is going to equip you with some basic information that you just need to implant at the back of your mind as you make your way through this carb cycling journey.

The Protection of the Thyroid

We already touched on how the thyroid hormone is a very important component for fat loss. A high level of thyroid hormones can help stimulate fat loss, but a low-carb diet can dramatically slow down the production of thyroid hormones. This detail is particularly important for women to keep in mind because they tend to have more sensitive thyroid behaviors and metabolism. During the low-carb days, it's important that women don't go overboard with their restrictions because it could negatively alter the production of thyroid hormones. Ideally, during low-carb days, women would still be consuming a little more than 50 grams of carbohydrates a day.

Female Insulin Sensitivity

When talking about the hormones that get affected by carbohydrate consumption, one must never forget about estrogen and progesterone. You might not have thought about this before, but your menstrual cycle can also dramatically impact the way that your body metabolizes the food that you consume. Depending on where you are on your menstrual cycle, it's either the carbs that you eat get processed more efficiently or they might end up being reserved as fat storage. This is why it would be better for you to somehow merge your carb cycling schedule with your menstrual cycle.

Normally, a woman's estrogen levels would be at their highest during the first two weeks of a menstrual cycle. During these initial two weeks, progesterone levels would also be at their lowest. What this means for dieting is that the body is more efficient at processing carbohydrates during these periods. In the luteal phase of a menstrual cycle (the last two weeks after ovulation), progesterone levels rise to a higher degree. This means that the body isn't going to be able to process carbohydrates all that well. This is a natural phenomenon that might be familiar to diabetic women. Typically, women with diabetes have to increase their dosage of insulin during the luteal phase of their menstrual cycle due to their blood sugar levels being relatively higher than usual.

So, what does this all mean for when you decide to start carb cycling?

Given that your menstrual cycles dictate your body's insulin levels, it's important that you time your carb cycles appropriately. To find the most success with carb cycling, it is advised that you reduce the amount of carbohydrates that you eat during the luteal phase or the last two weeks of your menstrual cycle. This is the period wherein your insulin sensitivity is going to be at its lowest, and it's important that you adjust your carb intake levels accordingly. So, given that you have to be very strict with your carb intake during your luteal phase, you have more liberty and freedom during the first two weeks of your cycle.

Of course, for a beginner, this might seem a little too vague or ambiguous for you. So, if you're looking for a real number that you can choose to work with, it would be best if you shoot for around 150 to 200 grams of carbohydrates every day for the first two weeks of your carb cycling. During the second week of the cycle, you even have the freedom to bump it up to around 220 to 250 grams of carbohydrates depending on your physical activity.

For the final two weeks of the cycle, this is where you have to start to taper your carb consumption significantly. You might want to consider dropping your carb intake to around a little over half of the amount that you were consuming during the initial two weeks. However, it's important that you don't overdo it by consistently going below 100 grams of carbs per day. This might impact your ability to conceive and also aggravate your thyroid issues.

Getting Fit for Women

As far as exercising is concerned, it shouldn't be something that you are wary of or be intimidated by. In fact, no matter what your gender, you should always make it a point to incorporate a healthy exercise routine into your daily life. Regular exercise is not only safe for everyone, but it's something that should be encouraged among all people. It's merely a matter of adopting an exercise routine or regimen that is well-suited for your lifestyle and biomechanical makeup. If you're doing carb cycling, then it's advisable for you to definitely incorporate exercise into your routine to maximize the effects of your diet.

Given that we've already talked about how your menstrual cycle can impact the effectiveness of your dieting, it shouldn't come as a surprise to you that it can affect the effectiveness of your training as well. To get straight to the point, during the initial two weeks of your cycle, you should engage in training that is more aerobic in nature. This means that your workouts should be performed at medium intensity, and they should be sustained for a relatively long period of time. Again, during your first two weeks, your carb intake is at your highest. This is why it's a good idea for you to push yourself with the length and duration of your workouts. It's not so much about increasing intensity. It's just about managing your energy well so that you are expending copious amounts of it over a sustained period. Don't be afraid to really push yourself as this is the phase of your cycle wherein your body is really primed to handle stressful physical conditions.

For the final two weeks of your cycle, this is where you want to consider just engaging in exercises that are more anaerobic in nature. Again, your carb intake is very low, and you might not have enough energy to sustain long and grueling training sessions. However, in order to compensate for the drop in workout durations, you have to make up for it with intensity. You should aim to get to around 80% to 90% of your maximum heart rate during these training periods. They don't have to last as long, but your training sessions have to leave you feeling like you gave it everything you've got in a short span of time. Some examples of anaerobic exercises are weightlifting, high intensity interval training, sprint intervals, and the like. Another added benefit of engaging in intense exercise sessions is that it helps sharpen your insulin sensitivity during this phase of your cycle. This means that you are able to burn and process fat more efficiently throughout the day even when you're no longer working out.

Mastering the Art of Cycle Syncing

All right, so a lot of important concepts have been laid out so far, and hopefully, they were able to provide you some deep insight into how your menstrual cycle affects your body. However, it can be very easy to just be overwhelmed by all of that info to the point that you end up forgetting some vital aspects of it. But in reality, it's all very simple. If you really want a more general overview of the important concepts behind syncing your carb and menstrual cycles, just remember that your typical menstrual cycle in relation to your carb cycle is made up of four different phases: menstrual, follicular, ovulatory, and luteal. The way that you eat and the way that you exercise should be dependent on which phase of the cycle you are currently in.

There are definitely some key concepts that you need to pay attention to with regards to syncing your dietary cycles and your menstrual cycles. And in order for you to really get the most out of your diet, you have to be willing to go the extra mile by paying close attention to all of the details. In order to systemize the planning process for you, it might be a good idea to take a phase-by-phase approach to discussing the ins and outs of cycle syncing.

Benefits of Cycle Syncing

If you're still in need of further convincing on why cycle syncing is going to serve you and your body well, then here are a few things that might incentivize you to really take this concept seriously. Aside from promoting weight loss and optimal athletic performance, carb cycling can also:

- minimize the effects of PMS or menstrual cramps
- decrease the chances of you getting hormonal acne

- balance your hormones after using a pill or IUD
- regulate your period if you have amenorrhea
- regulate your postpartum hormones
- minimize or eliminate the symptoms of PCOS
- optimize your body for conception

Foods to Avoid for Cycle Syncing

We've already discussed how there are certain foods that you should always try to have during certain phases of your cycle. However, before we get into the specifics of the food that you HAVE to eat, it's important to discuss the food that you have to eliminate altogether. Unfortunately, there are just certain popular food items out there that are loved by many but can wreak absolute chaos on hormone levels. Of course, depending on your age and fitness level, you might be able to get away with sneaking a few servings of these *banned* treats every once in a while. But for the most part, if you really want to make the most out of your diet, stay as strict as possible by avoiding these foods:

- processed and refined foods with non-natural ingredients
- white sugar
- margarine
- processed meats such as cold cuts and hot dogs
- canned goods
- deep-fried fast food
- hydrogenated oils
- soda
- high fructose corn syrup and other artificial sweeteners

Finding Your Phase

When it comes to cycle syncing, timing is everything. All of it hinges on you knowing which phase of your menstrual cycle you are in. If you are someone who has a regular cycle, then you stand to benefit from using an app that can help you track where you are. However, the general rule of thumb is that the first day of your menstrual cycle is also the day of your first big flow of blood. Things can get a little tricky when you have an irregular cycle. If you have an irregular cycle, it doesn't mean that you won't be able to reap the benefits of cycle syncing. Instead of relying on your menstrual cycle, you can use the lunar phases as a reference. If you haven't noticed, the lunar cycle also lasts for 28 days, much like a menstrual cycle. You can make use of various apps or internet sources to help you keep track of the lunar phases.

Menstrual Phase

The main thing that takes place on the first day of your menstrual phase is the shedding of the lining of your uterus. This takes place after your hormone levels drop, and this sends a signal to the tissues that are lining your uterus to shed and exit the body. In most cases, before the 7th day of the menstrual phase, the bleeding will have ceased. In the lead-up to this time, follicles are developed on the ovaries, and these contain eggs that are waiting to be fertilized.

But why does any of that information matter when it comes to plotting your diet?

This is because all of the hormonal changes taking place in your body during the menstrual phase are going to impact your energy levels dramatically. This is because your body will be depleted of estrogen at the start of the phase and will gradually rise up towards the end of it. You are also going to experience some iron deficiency as a result of all the blood that you're losing. Given that, you want to make sure that your diet is one that is rich in iron. Also, try consuming foods that help reduce inflammation to minimize the discomforts of menstruation.

So, when you're planning your diet for the menstrual phase, make sure to incorporate a lot of food that is warm and comforting. Go for a lot of soups, broths, casseroles, or stews that don't have too many harsh ingredients but are still filling and nutritious.

Follicular Phase

The follicular phase of the menstrual cycle typically lasts from days 7 to 14. It's during this phase wherein the estrogen and testosterone levels in the body will rise continuously while the linings of the uterus wall will start to thicken again. During the follicular phase, expect to feel somewhat energized, especially compared to how you were feeling in the menstrual phase. In this phase, you should take most of the energy that you're feeling to really go hard at the gym or wherever your workouts are. Really try to push yourself as this is usually the time of the month when you will be your strongest.

Typically, this is also going to be the phase where your body will be primed to burn up large amounts of calories. Don't be afraid to indulge in a lot of healthy carbohydrates, but also make sure that you are capitalizing on protein and fat intake as well. If you are a bodybuilder, then this is the time of the month for you to move some serious weight. And if you're putting the work in the gym, then make sure that you reward yourself with food. To be more specific, go for a lot of lean meats, healthy oils, fruits, and vegetables.

Ovulation Phase

After the follicular phase, the egg will travel down the fallopian tubes, making its way to the uterus. If the egg happens to meet sperm there, then the egg will become fertilized and travel down the tube even further to attach itself to the lining of the uterus. Coming from the highs of the follicular phase, you will experience a lot of grogginess and sluggishness here in the ovulation phase. You might also experience some bloating and it's possible that you will gain some weight during this period. However, you shouldn't worry much. It's probably just water weight as the result of the rising progesterone levels in your body.

Generally, you are going to want to focus on consuming a lot of fiber during this phase to ease any discomfort in your digestive system. Go for fruits and vegetables that are rich in fiber to aid your bowel movement. Also, it's very likely that your sugar level will drop during this phase. So, you want to make sure that you're still filling yourself up with a healthy dose of carbohydrates to balance your insulin levels out and keep yourself energized. However, avoid any carbohydrates that are too complex or strenuous to process such as wheats, grains, or pastas. For your training, stick to aerobic exercises that are performed at medium intensity. It's likely that you are going to burn way more calories during this phase with aerobic exercises.

Luteal Phase

The luteal phase is also the final phase of the menstrual cycle before the blood starts flowing again. During this phase, the uterus lining will really thicken itself up before it starts shedding itself in the menstrual phase. If the egg has not been fertilized by sperm, the estrogen and progesterone levels of the body will decrease, and this will signal the start of a new menstrual cycle. The egg will break away from the lining of the uterus, and it will also be shed during the next period.

Expect to feel really tired and moody during this phase. Your body is using up a lot of energy to gear up for a new menstrual cycle. As a result, there isn't really all that much energy left for you to do other things. Also, your serotonin levels will drop together with your estrogen. Remember that serotonin is a mood-balancing hormone. When your serotonin is compromised, it can be easy for you to feel overwhelmed by all of your feelings and emotions. Fortunately, exercise can help trigger the release of endorphins in your body, and this can help offset the dwindling levels of serotonin. After all, endorphins are known to be the natural happy hormones.

Also, since you don't have much energy to sustain long and grueling workouts, opt for shorter but more intense ones instead. This way, you are still getting the benefits of a full workout without having to use up too much of your stamina for it.

Final Thoughts

So as long as you remember those key points about the different phases of your menstrual cycle, you should do fine. Yes, it can be very complicated at the start to develop a plan that's going to work well for you. However, with more experience and experimentation, you will be able to drill your routine down to a tee. It's just a matter of staying patient and resilient with the diet. You shouldn't expect to get everything right on the first try. Make sure that you don't grow frustrated at the first signs of adversity. It's important that you stick with it and trust the process. Eventually, the results are going to come. You just can't rush and bypass the important aspects of the initial phases of carb cycling.

You might think that being a woman puts you at a disadvantage with your carb cycling because there are so many additional things that you need to keep track of. However, that isn't necessarily the case. In fact, you can use all of this extra knowledge and information to your advantage to really maximize the benefits of employing a carb cycling scheme for yourself.

Chapter 3:
Principles Behind Planning

We are very close to you getting to plot your own carb cycling plan. You have already been exposed to the many ways in which carb cycling is going to be different for you as compared to men. Of course, this new information might have complicated things a bit. But, at the very least, you are now armed with some of the knowledge that is necessary to make a more holistic and well-rounded plan for yourself. Again, remember that being a woman doesn't necessarily mean that you are at a disadvantage when it comes to your weight loss goals. It merely means that there are different things that you need to be keeping track of as far as variables and factors are concerned.

Now, it's time to tackle some concepts and principles that can be considered as commonalities between men and women. Again, we are very close to having you create your own plan. But before we get there, you have to familiarize yourself with a few important concepts and principles about the planning method. Remember, it's not just about randomly picking days where you consume large amounts of carbs or low amounts of carbs. It's also not just about randomly deciding on which number constitutes high and low consumption sizes either. There is a real mathematical science to it with rules that you need to adhere to if you want the diet to be effective.

Consider this chapter to be the final phase of the theoretical portion of this book. Soon, you are going to get a lot of practical tips and even a real opportunity to create your own plan for yourself. But first, it's very important that you really drill these important concepts and principles into your mind first. In this chapter, you will be given a very detailed breakdown of the principles of macro-counting and why it's important for you to do the math when determining your meal plan. Also, you will be briefed on some very basic principles that concern your developing a real diet plan for yourself. And at the end of this chapter, you will be given a sample meal plan that you can use to model your own diet plan after.

By the end of this chapter, you should be armed with all of the theoretical knowledge that you need to develop an effective carb cycling plan for yourself. You might be getting really fed up with a lot of these concepts, and that's understandable. However, you must also accept that losing serious weight over a sustainable period isn't just a matter of you winging it and hoping for the best. The reason that a lot of people struggle with losing weight is because it's a difficult endeavor, and it requires a lot of attention to detail. You need to have the patience that is necessary for you to gather all of the information that you need in order for you to be as educated as possible prior to putting things into practice.

Breaking the Cycle Down According to Macros

This may not necessarily be the first time that you've encountered the idea of counting *macros* for dieting. In fact, there is a very popular diet plan called IIFYM, or *If It Fits Your Macros,* and a lot of people actually swear by this dieting philosophy. This method of dieting is also known as flexible dieting as it doesn't really disallow people from certain foods. Rather, it limits one from overindulging in particular food types. This might all seem really vague right now, but you'll understand it more along the way.

What Are Macros?

First, we need to talk more in-depth about what macros are before we start talking about how you can count them and why they factor into your carb cycles. Macros or *macronutrients* are the three major nutrients that make up the bulk of the food that you eat on a daily basis to nourish yourself. The three macronutrients are protein, carbs, and fat. Each macro is going to have a corresponding caloric value, and they all serve different purposes in nourishing the human body. There are some foods that will have generous doses of each macronutrient. However, most of the time, a food item will only be biased towards just one or two macros. For example, most meats are heavy in protein and fat. Wheats and grains are mostly loaded with carbohydrates. Oils are almost exclusively made up of fat. In order for your body to function optimally, you need appropriate doses of each macronutrient. So, let's break down the three macros, shall we?

Carbohydrates. No, they're not the enemy. Forget everything that you've been told about carbs. A lot of the time, when the mainstream media tries to come up with marketing campaigns to scare people into getting fit, they depict images of overweight people munching down on carb-rich food like ice cream, doughnuts, pizza, and whatnot. Sure, it's true that an overindulgence in carbohydrates can make a person fat. But you can also say the same for any other macronutrient as well. There really isn't much sense in singling out carbohydrates as a macronutrient that needs to be avoided at all costs. Remember, weight loss or weight gain is all a matter of calories going in or out of the body. And a single gram of carbohydrates is going to carry around 4 calories. One gram of carbohydrates carries the same caloric value as a single gram of protein. And yet, carbohydrates are hailed as the devil, and protein is propped up to be *the* health macro. Keep in mind that carbs are responsible for fueling the body with energy. You wouldn't be able to work out at the gym or train on the track at an optimal level if you didn't have any carbs in your system. When you eat carbs, your body processes them into glucose, which serves as the source of your body's energy to do everything that it needs to function properly. However, when there is excess energy leftover, it then gets converted as stored fat. This is the reason why overconsumption of carbs is bad and why this macro often gets a bad rap in the fitness community.

Fats. Next up, there are fats. Fat is actually another macronutrient that is known to have a bad rap in the fitness community. When carb-heavy foods like doughnuts or chocolates aren't being demonized in mainstream media, it's usually fat-heavy food like fried chicken, cheeseburgers, and fast food items. However, unlike carbohydrates, there is some validity to the demonization of fats due to its caloric values. A single gram of fat carries a whopping 9 calories. But that doesn't mean that fat is a macro that should be avoided at all costs. Again, it's just a matter of managing the consumption of fat so as to not fall into the trap of overindulgence. Fats are vital to the normal and healthy function of a human body. Contrary to what most people are led to believe, eating fat won't necessarily translate to you also getting fat. This myth has already been debunked by the success of the keto diet, a fat-centric diet that stimulates weight loss. However, there are just certain fat-heavy foods that have little nutritional value and might lead to the surplus of calories which can eventually lead to weight gain. Examples of unhealthy fat sources are vegetable oils, margarine, and fast food, which are very bad for the body. But on the other side of the spectrum, there are healthy fat sources like avocados, coconut oil, nuts, nut butters, and more that offer a lot of nutritional value. Fats like these are responsible for making sure that the body is able to efficiently absorb and process nutrients in the body. On top of that, fats aid in hormone and body temperature regulation as well.

Protein. Lastly, there is protein. This is the macronutrient that is most often heralded as the ideal poster child for health and wellness. And it's really not all that hard to see why. Regardless of whatever your fitness goals might be, it's always important that you incorporate a generous allocation of protein into your diet. As with carbohydrates, proteins only have 4 calories for every gram. This means that you have more liberty to eat more of it without having to worry about going into a caloric surplus. Also, this is the macronutrient that is responsible for building the muscular cells and tissues in your body. This is precisely the reason why protein is the go-to macro for serious athletes like weightlifters, bodybuilders, runners, and more. Protein is a macronutrient that is most commonly found in meat, beans, seafood, and poultry to name a few.

Determining Your TDEE or Total Daily Energy Expenditure

Now, just because you know what macros are doesn't mean that you can get started on determining how much of them you need to eat. There is one last step that you need to perform before you can calculate your recommended macro numbers. You must first find out what your *TDEE* or total daily energy expenditure is. Don't worry. It isn't going to require you to do a lot of heavy math. In fact, it's merely a matter of inputting some values into a calculator that you can find online and have the computer do the work for you. The calculator found at **https://tdeecalculator.net/** is a perfect one that you can use. Essentially, the TDEE is a determination of how many calories you are using up every day based on your age, body composition, and level of your physical activity.

Your body typically has a base metabolic rate or a BMR. This is essentially how many calories your body will burn while it's at rest. Your BMR is computed based on your physical composition and your age. However, the TDEE is a more comprehensive evaluation of how many calories you are burning every day as it takes into consideration your level of physical activity as well. The reason why it's important for you to learn your TDEE is because it gives you a solid number to work with when figuring out the distribution of your macros.

So, whatever result you get for your TDEE calculation is essentially the number of calories that you need to eat every day to maintain your weight. In order for you to lose or gain weight, you need to get in either a caloric deficit or surplus, respectively. One pound of fat approximates to around 3,500 calories. So, if you want to lose one pound of fat, you are going to have to get into a caloric deficit of 3,500 calories. Obviously, it wouldn't be practical for regular folk to be getting into a deficit of 3,500 calories every single day. This is only a number that is achievable for the highest-level athletes who train multiple hours in a day. For the most part, people should only shoot for a caloric deficit of around 500 to 1,000 calories per day. This should enable you to lose 1 to 2 pounds a week. So, let's say that based on your TDEE calculation, you are burning 2,200 calories every day. If you restrict yourself to eating just 1,200 calories per day, you will eventually lose 2 pounds within a span of a week. However, take note that this is not an exact science and that there is a chance that you will lose more or less weight than is expected. There really is no way that you can accurately gauge just how many calories you burn on any given day. But the TDEE calculator should give you a fairly good idea of a ballpark number that you can use as a guide. Also, make sure your target daily caloric deficit doesn't fall outside the 500 to 1,000 calorie range. Sure, you can try to exceed that if you're looking to lose a huge amount of weight quickly. However, that wouldn't be a healthy or a sustainable way to go about weight loss.

Calculating Your Macros

Again, calories don't necessarily tell the whole story. Sure, in essence, you would be able to lose weight by merely tracking your calories alone. But a more holistic approach to health and wellness requires you to actively and accurately track your macros. However, tracking your macros requires you to know your TDCI or target daily caloric intake. You will learn more about how to compute your ideal TDCI later on in the book., You need to use your TDCI as a foundation to build your macro consumption breakdown. If we go back to the example that was used in the previous step, you might limit yourself to just 1,200 calories per day so that you can lose 2 pounds a week. So, based on that, your TDCI would be 1,200 calories. The breakdown of your macros should be based on this number.

Ideally, this is how you want to distribute your macros:

Your carbs should make up around 40-60% of your calories. Fats should make up 20-30% of calories. And protein should make up 20-40% of calories. Earlier, we learned that every gram of each macro is going to carry a corresponding caloric value. Carbs and proteins have 4 calories each for every gram, and fats have 9 calories for every gram. To determine how many grams of each macro you need to eat, you just have to divide the caloric allocation you have for each macro by its corresponding caloric value. Don't worry, all of this might be a little difficult to imagine for now, so let's try to put these formulas to work.

Let's say, that based on the recommended caloric allocations, you have decided to break down your macros into 50% carbs, 30% protein, and 20% fat. So, based on those values together with your TDCI, this is how the distribution of your macros should look:

Total Carbs = 1,200 * 0.5 = 600 / 4 = 150 grams

Total Protein = 1,200 * 0.3 = 360 / 4 = 90 grams

Total Fat = 1,200 * 0.2 = 240 / 9 = 26.7 grams

Of course, this is just a general recommendation and example of what someone's daily macro distribution and consumption could look like. However, as mentioned, this book isn't about to give you a cookie-cutter recommendation. If you are reading this book, you are a woman who wants to lose weight through carb cycling. With that, there are specific numbers that you should be hitting in order for you to achieve your goals. And as mentioned, when you are carb cycling, you aren't eating the same amount of carbs every day.

Ideal Macros for High and Low Days

So, now you have the formula for computing your macros. It wasn't all that hard, right? If the manual computations really trouble you, feel free to make use of various tools or apps that you can find on your phone or on the internet to help you out. In any case, knowing how to compute your ideal macros is only part of the battle. Now, you have to figure out how to adjust your macro distribution based on your high- and low-carb days.

Just for a quick refresher, when you are carb cycling, you are essentially giving yourself intervals for your carb consumption. There are certain days in which you should be taking relatively high amounts of carbohydrates, and there should be days where you are taking low amounts. Determining which days of the week should be your high or low ones is a topic that will be discussed in the latter parts of this chapter. For now, you have to figure out how you're going to compute your macros relative to your high and low days. The example that was given previously was merely a format for someone who was tracking macros without going through carb cycling. If we take that same example and apply carb cycling principles to it, this is how it would look:

For high-carb days, you want to make sure that this is where you really insert a bulk of your carb consumption throughout the week. However, all of the same principles of macro calculation apply. It's merely a matter of adjusting target values. In the previous example, only 50% of the TDCI was accounted for by carbohydrates. Maybe, on high-carb days, you can bump that number up to 55% or even 60%. Your decision will depend on your level of physical activity or on whatever works for you. So, since you bumped your carb allocation up to 55%, doesn't that mean that you would be exceeding your TDCI? Yes, that is true. This is why one or both of the other macros should adjust. Of course, you can adjust the numbers based on your own personal preference. However, if you're a beginner and you don't know how to go about those adjustments, the general rule of thumb is that when your carbs go up, your fat should go down, and vice-versa. The protein consumption should remain relatively consistent on both high- and low-carb days. So, on high-carb days, if you're increasing consumption of carbs by around 5%, then that means you need to take 5% of calories away from your fat consumption. Based on the given example, the new macro distribution of your high-carb days should look like this:

Total Carbs = 1,200 * 0.55 = 660 / 4 = 165 grams

Total Protein = 1,200 * 0.3 = 360 / 4 = 90 grams

Total Fat = 1,200 * 0.15 = 180/ 9 = 20 grams

Again, this is just an example, and it's okay if your plan for high-carb days doesn't exactly look like this. This is merely an illustration of how you would adjust your macro distribution for high-carb days. Now, for your low-carb days, it's important that you really limit your carbs as much as possible. However, as has been previously mentioned, for women, it's important that you never consistently stray too far away from the 100 gram-threshold for minimum carb consumption. With the way that your body is wired, it's important that you don't deprive yourself of carbs too much in order for your body to function properly. So, if on high-carb days, you are looking to increase your average carb consumption by 5%, maybe it would be okay for you to decrease your carbs by 10% on low-carb days. Let's see what that looks like:

Total Carbs = 1,200 * 0.40 = 480/ 4 = 120 grams

Total Protein = 1,200 * 0.3 = 360 / 4 = 90 grams

Total Fat = 1,200 * 0.3 = 360 / 9 = 40 grams

With this example, you are staying within the safe zone for minimal carb consumption as a woman. However, feel free to push the envelope even further if you're up for the challenge. Try to gradually lower your carb consumption on low-carb days and see how it works for you. If your body responds well and you're feeling fine, then keep it up. If you start feeling sluggish and too tired over an extended period of time, it might be a sign that you're not eating enough. So, again, it's important for you to really listen to your body.

Let's try to change the values a little bit as we illustrate another example. Imagine that you are a woman whose goal is to eat just 1,500 calories a day. For high-carb days, you have decided that you will be eating 60% carbs, 20% protein, and 20% fat. For low-carb days, you think that you would be able to handle 35% carbs, 30% protein, and 35% fat.

For high-carb days, this is how the computations should play out:

Total Carbs = 1,500 * 0.6 = 900 / 4 = 225 grams

Total Protein = 1,500 * 0.2 = 300 / 4 = 75 grams

Total Fat = 1,500 * 0.2 = 300 / 9 = 33.3 grams

For low-carb days, this is how much you would be eating:

Total Carbs = 1,500 * 0.35 = 525 / 4 = 131.25 grams

Total Protein = 1,500 * 0.3 = 500 / 4 = 125 grams

Total Fat = 1,500 * 0.35 = 525 / 9 = 58.3 grams

There you have it. Hopefully, you have a much clearer picture by now of how you would compute your macros for your high and low days. Yes, it might feel like a lot of work. However, most of this kind of work is only done at the start. Remember, you have been warned that carb cycling is going to have a very meticulous planning process. But at the very least, if you develop a plan that works and you manage to stick to it, you are undoubtedly going to yield favorable results.

How To Make a Diet Plan

Now, we've discussed all of the annoying numerical aspects of making your diet plan. You're probably all fed up with all of these numbers and computations by now. Don't worry. That aspect of the planning and preparation process is over. Now, it's time to really develop your plan and figure out how to plot your low- and high-carb days. Of course, given that you are the architect of your own plan, this is where you have more freedom to really experiment and play around with what is going to work best for you. There are many different possible approaches that you could take to making your carb cycling plan. Some people choose to alternate on a daily basis. There are those who go a few days on high and a few days on low. There are also those who take a weekly interval approach to cycling. Again, it really depends on what kind of person you are and the lifestyle that you have.

However, for you, the reader, a woman who is looking to lose weight, we need to take a more specialized approach to determining your carb cycle. In a previous chapter, we talked about how it would be ideal for you to synchronize your carb and menstrual cycles in order to make the most out of your diet. So, we will integrate those principles into making your plan. Also, make sure that you incorporate some level of exercise into your plan as well. Hopefully, if you are reading, you are still physically able to move athletically to the point that you are capable of exercising or working out. It doesn't matter if you have a very low level of fitness. So as long as you have the capacity to move, you should be exercising. Heck, even a quick internet search will show you videos of disabled or differently-abled people doing some of the most intense workouts you will ever see. There's no excuse there. If you are serious about losing weight, then you need to exercise.

This is going to be a sample diet and exercise plan that you can use if you are looking to synchronize your menstrual cycle together with your diet and fitness regimen. Again, remember that you are going to want to shoot for high-carb days during the first two weeks of the cycle and then taper off towards the final two weeks. If you need a refresher on this, feel free to return back to the second chapter discussing how your menstrual cycle impacts your insulin sensitivity levels. In any case, here is a recommended carb cycling diet plan that takes into consideration your level of exercise output and menstrual cycle for a woman who is eating 1,500 calories per day.

Day 1: low carbs (125 grams) with high volume training

Day 2: high carbs (230 grams) with high volume training

Day 3: high carbs (200 grams) with high volume training

Day 4: low carbs (115 grams) with minimal training/active recovery

Day 5: high carbs (220 grams) with high volume training

Day 6: high carbs (220 grams) with high intensity training

Day 7: low carbs (1oo grams) with minimal training/active recovery

Day 8: medium-high (180 grams) carbs with high intensity training

Day 9: high carbs (200 grams) with high volume training

Day 10: high carbs (215 grams) with high volume training

Day 11: high carbs (220 grams) with high volume training

Day 12: high carbs (200 grams) with high intensity training

Day 13: low carbs (115 grams) with minimal training/active recovery

Day 14: high carbs (195 grams) with high volume training

Day 15: medium-high (180 grams) carbs with high intensity training

Day 16: low carbs (125 grams) with high intensity training

Day 17: low carbs (100 grams) with high intensity training

Day 18: low carbs (130 grams) with minimal training/active recovery

Day 19: low carbs (120 grams) with high intensity training

Day 20: low carbs (125 grams) with moderate intensity training

Day 21: low carbs (125 grams) with minimal training/active recovery

Day 22: low carbs (140 grams) with moderate intensity training

Day 23: low carbs (120 grams) with moderate intensity training

Day 24: low carbs (125 grams) with minimal training/active recovery

Day 25: medium carbs (185 grams) with high intensity training

Day 26: low carbs (130 grams) with high intensity training

Day 27: low carbs (125 grams) with high intensity training

Day 28: low carbs (120 grams) with minimal training/active recovery

Again, this is merely a sample plan that you can choose to adopt for yourself. Of course, since this is your diet plan, only you can determine if it works for you or not. Don't be afraid to fine-tune this plan as you go to better suit your lifestyle. Remember that a lot of what makes a diet sustainable is dependent on whether the dieter enjoys executing it or not. This book might serve as an authority figure or valuable resource in helping you shape your path, but it's still ultimately your own path. There is no *one way* to achieve weight loss for women through carb cycling. There is plenty of room for experimentation and trial-and-error here. Feel free to tweak this recommended plan however you see fit.

Sample Weekly Meal Plan

Of course, it's not enough that this book advises you on which days you should be having high carbs and low carbs. You need to gain better insight into what the meals for those days should look like as well. For this part of the chapter, we are going to look into some concrete meal plans that you can use for your high- and low-carb distributions. For the purposes of this sample meal plan, we will assume the following format for carb cycling over a seven-day cycle:

Low-High-High-Low-High-High-Low

Day 1: Low-Carb Day

Breakfast: 4-Egg and Cheese Omelette with Toast Slices

Calories: 383 kcal, Carbs: 36 g, Fat: 17 g, Protein: 21 g

Lunch: Zucchini and Walnut Salad

Calories: 595 kcal, Carbs: 8 g, Fat: 58 g, Protein: 9 g

Snacks: Almond Milkshake

Calories: 264 kcal, Carbs: 20 g, Fat: 16 g, Protein: 14 g

Dinner: Turkey Sandwich on Whole Wheat

Calories: 241 kcal, Carbs: 36 g, Fat: 4.5 g, Protein: 15.5 g

Day 2: High-Carb Day

Breakfast: Baked Mushroom and Egg with Chicken and Multigrain Rice

Calories: 600 kcal, Carbs: 47 g, Fat: 24 g, Protein: 47 g

Lunch: Peanut Orange Chicken with Vegetables and Rice

Calories: 602 kcal, Carbs: 47 g, Fat: 24 g, Protein: 50 g

Snacks: Peanut Butter Sandwich on Wheat Bread

Calories: 327 kcal, Carbs: 30 g, Fat: 18 g, Protein: 15 g

Dinner: Sweet and Spicy Beef Bowl

Calories: 459 kcal, Carbs: 45 g, Fat: 11 g, Protein: 40 g

Day 3: High-Carb Day

Breakfast: Peanut Butter Banana Oatmeal with Egg and Pulled Pork

Calories: 603 kcal, Carbs: 47 g, Fat: g, Protein: 49 g

Lunch: Slow-Cooked Chicken and Rice Casserole

Calories: 380 kcal, Carbs: 36 g, Fat: 11 g, Protein: 36 g

Snacks: Multigrain Bread with Olive Oil

Calories: 257 kcal, Carbs: 22.6 g, Fat: 16.2 g, Protein: 7 g

Dinner: Turkey Sandwich on Whole Wheat

Calories: 241 kcal, Carbs: 36 g, Fat: 4.5 g, Protein: 15.5 g

Day 4: Low-Carb Day

Breakfast: Cream Cheese Pancakes

Calories: 344 kcal, Carbs: 3 g, Fat: 29 g, Protein: 17 g

Lunch: Turkey Sandwich on Whole Wheat

Calories: 241 kcal, Carbs: 36 g, Fat: 4.5 g, Protein: 15.5 g

Snacks: Low-Carb Deviled Eggs

Calories: 163 kcal, Carbs: 0.5 g, Fat: 15 g, Protein: 7 g

Dinner: Fried Kale and Broccoli Salad

Calories: 1,022 kcal, Carbs: 13 g, Fat: 94 g, Protein: 22 g

Day 5: High-Carb Day

Breakfast: Fruity Oatmeal Bowl (High Carb)

Calories: 348 kcal, Carbs: 59 g, Fat: 10 g, Protein:7 g

Lunch: Moroccan Couscous with Flank Steak

Calories: 371 kcal, Carbs: 41 g, Fat: 9 g, Protein: 32 g

Snacks: Multigrain Bread with Olive Oil

Calories: 257 kcal, Carbs: 22.6 g, Fat: 16.2 g, Protein: 7 g

Dinner: Slow-Cooked Chicken and Rice Casserole

Calories: 380 kcal, Carbs: 36 g, Fat: 11 g, Protein: 36 g

Day 6: High-Carb Day

Breakfast: Cream Cheese Pancakes

Calories: 344 kcal, Carbs: 3 g, Fat: 29 g, Protein: 17 g

Lunch: Spicy Avocado Chicken Salad Wrap

Calories: 534 kcal, Carbs: 49 g, Fat: 18 g, Protein: 47 g

Snacks: Peanut Butter Sandwich on Wheat Bread

Calories: 327 kcal, Carbs: 30 g, Fat: 18 g, Protein: 15

Dinner: Slow-Cooked Chicken and Rice Casserole

Calories: 380 kcal, Carbs: 36 g, Fat: 11 g, Protein: 36 g

Day 7: Low-Carb Day

Breakfast: Keto Coconut Porridge

Calories: 486 kcal, Carbs: 4 g, Fat: 49 g, Protein: 9 g

Lunch: Zucchini and Walnut Salad

Calories: 595 kcal, Carbs: 8 g, Fat: 58 g, Protein: 9 g

Snacks: 1 oz of Almonds

Calories: 163 kcal, Carbs: 12 g, Fat: 2 g, Protein: 11 g

Dinner: Salad in a Jar

Calories: 876 kcal, Carbs: 11 g, Fat: 76 g, Protein: 27 g

Final Thoughts

Again, these are just some very rough concepts that you can choose to adopt for your own personal diet plan. Regardless, all of the principles are laid out here, and they should serve as the foundation for your diet. At the end of the day, you are really going to have to get in there and make a few adjustments to better suit your own personal needs and goals. If you are looking to really follow this meal plan, you will find the recipes for these food items in another chapter towards the end of this book.

Author's Note

So, are you enjoying the book so far? Maybe you should take a quick breather and gather your thoughts for a bit. A lot of very deep and important concepts have already been covered, and you may need to take some time to reflect on them. Hopefully, you will have gained some profound insight into carb cycling by now. As an author, it would make me really happy to know that my words have added some degree of value to your life. In my line of work, reviews are really hard to come by, and they can really help push my career forward so that I can come up with more meaningful content like this to help you and other people as well.

With that, I wish you could just take the time right now to write a brief review of this book on any book-selling platform (Amazon, for example). It doesn't have to be anything too complicated or anything. It just has to be honest. Any time that you spend to write a review would be greatly appreciated by me and many writers like myself. Thank you so much for reading this book and taking the time to write a review for it. It really means a lot to me. Now, onwards to the rest of the book!

Chapter 4:
Create Your Own Plan

Not to hype this chapter up, but everything that you have read so far in this book has led to this. It's now time for you to create your own diet plan for yourself. Consider this to be the output of everything that you've been working hard to learn up to this point. Yes, gaining knowledge and proficiency in theory is all well and good. It's important. However, none of that will be of value unless you are able to apply your lessons to your everyday life. And this chapter is going to guide you throughout that process.

It can't be emphasized enough that the planning and preparation phases of carb cycling might be the most important. It doesn't matter how strictly you execute your plan if it's a faulty one to begin with. When you seriously want to get into carb cycling, it's vital that you really take the time to sit down and develop a plan that is foolproof. So, before we get right into the thick of things with this chapter, a few reminders are warranted. Then, you should have some kind of documentation device ready as we proceed to the latter parts of this chapter where you will start developing your own plan.

It's not enough that this book just supplies you a comprehensively laid out plan that you can follow to the tee. Remember that this book's author has no knowledge of what kind of lifestyle you lead, how many hours you work, what level of fitness you have, and other such details. There are too many variables that need to be taken into consideration, and it's only you who has knowledge of those things. All that this book can provide you is a rough sketch or outline of the drawing that you need to finish. You just have to do the proper shading and coloring at this point.

Of course, you can always choose to go the easy route and merely adopt some kind of ready-made outline that is available online. A quick internet search will present you with a myriad of ready-made options that you can choose to follow on your own. You might be able to find success in it and you might not. Whatever the case, know that taking the time to really pay attention to all the details of fine-tuning your diet to your lifestyle will serve you better in the long run.

Think of your diet like it's a dress. When you go shopping for dresses, it's a lot of fun, right? You see different dresses that are fit for differently sized people, and they come in all sorts of shapes and colors. There are some dresses that you admire, but they don't fit you. And there are some dresses that might fit you really well, but you aren't really a fan of particular details like its colors or stitch patterns. But eventually, you are bound to find a dress that will be *okay* and do the job. You buy it and you look good in it. You make it work. But ultimately, you know that the dress isn't *perfect*.

That's the shopping equivalent of just taking a ready-made carb cycling pattern online and applying it to your own life. Sure, you can probably find something that you like and that will grant you some success. But buying a ready-to-wear dress is nothing compared to visiting a proper designer and creating a dress from scratch. By getting a dress designed specifically for you, you are granted the opportunity to pore over every single detail. You will have a say in the crafting of the dress from the start right to the finish. And the end product is bound to be something that you're happy with… all because you took the time to take a more active role in the planning and design process.

Think of this chapter as you are chatting with your designer about your dream dress. Except now, we're talking about your dream diet. Yes, there are certain rules and principles that you have to follow. And a lot of them have already been laid out here in this book. At this point, it's just a matter of taking everything that you learned and putting it all to paper (or jot it down on your phone if you're a techier person). Again, there is a lot of upside to decisively being the one who makes your diet plan from scratch. And if you're up for that challenge, this chapter is going to meticulously guide you through that process with a streamlined series of steps that you can follow to a tee.

But first... a few reminders.

Things to Remember When Making Your Own Diet Plan

Before we jump into the crafting of your specialized diet plan, there are a few things that you need to keep in mind first. Consider this segment of the chapter to be a short rehashing of everything that you have learned so far. It's important that you keep these guiding principles to heart so that you don't have to second-guess yourself throughout the entire process.

There Are Many Different Factors to Consider When Deciding on High and Low Intervals

When deciding on which days to designate as high-carb or low-carb days, there are a myriad of different factors that you need to consider. However, in order to simplify things for you, here are a few principles that you need to keep in mind:

- The heavier you are or bigger your current body mass, the more calories you are burning. So, you have a higher threshold for carb consumption than those who are smaller than you.
- On the days that you don't work out, you are burning fewer calories. So, it would be best if you designate these days as your low-carb days as well. This will help prevent weight gain even when you're not exercising.
- The more drastic your goals are, then the more drastic your carb cuts have to be. If you want to lose a large amount of weight in a short amount of time, then you need to seriously cut back on your calories. On high-carb days, make sure that you don't overindulge. On low-carb days, keep the numbers as low as you possibly can with your carb consumption.

- When your training for a particular day is aerobic in nature, feel free to have a high-carb day. Just make sure that your workouts are long enough for you to completely deplete your converted glucose. If your training day is more anaerobic or intense in nature, you will be able to get by with having a low-carb day.

- If you are training for a competition, be sure to factor your schedule into your diet plan. If you are training for a marathon, you will want to gradually increase your high-carb days as the competition nears. However, if you are training as a bodybuilder, you will want to have more low-carb days as you near the date of competition.

Carb Cycling Isn't the Same as Keto

While both dietary philosophies have you cutting down on carbs significantly to a certain degree, they don't necessarily trigger the same kind of processes in your body. With keto, you cut down on carbohydrates so that your body enters a ketogenic state. What this means is that your body has recognized a shortage of carbohydrates and has to search for alternative sources of energy. To do this, the body takes the fat reserves of the body and triggers the production of ketones in your liver. These ketones are then converted into the energy that is needed to fuel your body. By doing this, the body goes into an ultra-fat-burning mode in an effort to keep up with its own caloric demands.

On the other hand, with carb cycling, achieving ketosis isn't necessarily the end goal. Ultimately, the goal of carb cycling is to strengthen a body's insulin sensitivity while also achieving a caloric deficit in order to facilitate weight loss. Some of the side effects of carb cycling also include improved athletic performance and optimized digestive function.

Carb Cycling Is Different for Women than It Is for Men

This is the whole point of this book. Carb cycling is a process that can work for both men and women. However, there have to be different approaches for each gender. This is due to the fact that the hormonal makeup of men and women is fundamentally different. Keep in mind that the body's ability to burn fat is largely dependent on the state of one's hormone levels as well. When a carb cycling plan is not optimized for hormonal imbalances, then it might not be as effective as it should be.

It Would Be Best to Sync Carb and Menstrual Cycles

Studies have shown that a woman's hormone levels are heavily influenced by her menstrual cycle. So, in order to make the most out of a carb cycling dietary scheme, it is best to synchronize the carb cycle together with a woman's menstrual cycle. If you have irregular cycles, you can always opt to just synchronize your carb cycle with the lunar cycle instead.

On High-Carb Days, Eat Little Fat… and Vice-Versa

Ideally, you should aim for the same number of calories every day for you to lose weight. However, the makeup of your macro distribution should differ depending on whether you have a low-carb or a high-carb day. Regardless of whether you have a low-carb or high-carb day, your protein consumption should remain relatively consistent all throughout. The two macronutrients that you need to drastically adjust over the course of a cycle are your carbs and your fats. On high-carb days, make sure that you eat less fat. On low-carb days, eat more fat to make sure that you meet your daily caloric targets.

Don't Overcomplicate Things

Don't overcomplicate things. When you're developing your plan, there really is no need to make things more complicated than they already are. It's really just a matter of figuring out what days would better serve as low-carb or high-carb days. The math shouldn't be all that complicated either. All of the formulas have been laid out for you. You just have to input the values yourself and develop a plan around that. If all else fails, just remember KISS - keep it simple, sweetheart.

Step-by-Step Guide to Making Your Carb Cycling Plan

Do you have a pen and paper ready? It's time for you to start making your own carb cycling plan. Are you excited? You should be. This is a very important step that you are taking towards becoming the best and healthiest version of yourself. However, before you actually start putting your pen to paper, it's important to manage your expectations first. Be conscious of the fact that it's possible that the plan you come up with right now isn't necessarily going to give you the results that you want. Sometimes, you might not be losing as much weight as you want. In some instances, you might not even be losing weight at all. And in some rare cases, you might even find yourself gaining weight instead. If that's the case, don't give up. It's okay to be frustrated, but you shouldn't give up on the process entirely. Try to reassess your plan and make a few adjustments wherever you can. Ultimately, you shouldn't shy away from revisiting your plan in the future and tweaking things to make sure that your evolving needs are constantly being met.

With that said, let's proceed to the first step…

Step 1: Know Your Vital Statistics

First of all, you need to know your vital statistics. Obviously, this diet is a solution to a problem. You want to lose weight because you think that there is a problem with the current makeup of your body. However, it's not enough that you just think that you're overweight. You need to familiarize yourself with the numbers behind your body composition. At the very least, you should at least know how much you weigh before you start dieting. The number on the scale might not necessarily tell the whole story, but it definitely says a lot. Next, you must also know your

BMI or body mass index. There are those who will say that the BMI is an outdated measure of fitness and that it should be obsolete by now. And there is some truth to that. However, it can still serve as a somewhat accurate gauge of fitness for some people. If you really want to take things to another level, you can also get yourself measured for body fat percentage, VO2 max, and other health tests. The more you know about your body, then the better position you will be in to know what kind of work awaits you.

Step 2: Establish Your Goals

After step one, you should already have a good sense of where you are as far as your health and fitness levels are concerned. From this, you should be able to gather information on your potential points of improvement or problem area. For example, you might learn from your vital statistics that you are overweight and that you are at risk for heart disease, diabetes, or even cancer. So, you set a goal for yourself to lose a certain amount of weight just to make sure that you minimize your risk of contracting such complications. Perhaps you are already a relatively lean person, but you really want to try to chisel your body to allow your muscles to really shine. In order to do so, you have to lower your body fat percentage. Whatever the case, establishing a goal is very important. Your goal is going to serve as your *why* in everything that you do. This should be your primary mover and motivator to get the job done with your diet and training. Consider your goals to be your North Star. They are your guiding light. You can't just diet for the hell of it. In order to get anything substantial done in life, you must always be structured and purposeful with your actions.

Step 3: Set Your Training Regimen

This might be the step that a lot of you are going to show some level of hesitation with. This is especially true if you haven't really been athletic in your life. That's okay. It's normal to not be happy about the idea of having to develop a consistent training regimen. However, in order for you to really make the most out of your carb cycling diet, you have to be willing to exercise. The diet isn't going to work the way that it's supposed to if you don't take the time to incorporate exercise into your daily routine.

Of course, you don't have to train to be a superstar athlete or anything. You don't have to make it a point to spend hours on end at the gym. Experts say that the recommended time that you should be working out is at least 3 to 5 times a week for around 30 minutes to 1 hour per session. Ideally, you would elevate your heart rate to around 60% to 80% of your max heart rate during these sessions. This way, you are building cardiovascular strength, and you are also burning calories to facilitate weight loss at the same time.

Step 4: Find Your Total Daily Energy Expenditure (TDEE)

Another reason why you had to figure out your workout routine was so that you could have a more accurate gauge of your TDEE, or total daily energy expenditure. In order for you to figure out how much food you need to eat every day to lose weight, you have to figure out how many calories you are burning on a daily basis first. Now, keep in mind that different people burn different amounts of calories every day. There are plenty of factors that can help influence a body's metabolic output, such as body mass, level of physical activity, and age.

Also, there really is no accurate way for you to gauge how many calories you are burning. However, there is a calculator that you can make use of online to give you a rough estimate or a ballpark figure of how many calories you lose every day. This step has already been laid out in detail for you in a previous chapter of this book.

Step 5: Find Your Total Daily Caloric Intake

Once you've found out your TDEE, it's now time for you to compute your total daily caloric intake. This is where you begin to incorporate your goals, your vital stats, and your TDEE. All of the steps that preceded this one were vital for this particular computation. In this step, you have to figure out how much food you SHOULD be consuming every day in order for you to lose the amount of weight that you want. This is also called your total daily caloric intake or TDCI.

Keep in mind that a single pound of fat is going to equate to 3,500 calories. So, to put it simply, if you want to lose 1 pound, you need to burn 3,500 calories. If you want to lose 2 pounds, you have to burn 7,000 calories and so on...

So, to compute for your total daily caloric intake, you just have to take your TDEE and decrease it by around 500 to 1,000 depending on how drastic you want your weight loss to be. Of course, the safest and most sustainable caloric deficit for you to take every day would be just 500 to 1,000 calories. However, there are some people who are capable of fast-tracking their weight loss by exceeding that threshold. If you are an experienced fitness enthusiast, maybe you can experiment with going higher. However, if you are just a beginner, try your best to just stay within this range.

If you are consistently generating a deficit of 500 calories per day over the span of a week, then you will have lost at least 1 pound within that same span. So, assuming that you have a TDEE of 2,300 calories and you are looking to lose 1 pound in a week, that means you would have to consume 1,800 calories per day. Take note that your TDEE is going to change as you get slimmer and leaner. So, as a result, you might have to adjust your TDCI values along the way as well.

Step 6: Calculate Your Macros for High- and Low-Carb Days

This is a step that has already been discussed exhaustively in the previous chapter. If you need a quick refresher, feel free to go back and read about it. However, the general rule of thumb here is that you shouldn't try to shoot for anything too far below 100 grams of carbohydrates even on your low-carb days. As a woman, you still need these carbs in order for your body to function healthily and properly. Remember, carb cycling is merely about limiting and managing your carb intake properly. It's not about eliminating carbohydrates altogether.

Also, in addition to that, don't forget to keep in mind that your protein consumption should remain relatively consistent on both your high- and low-carb days. It's typically with your intake of fats and carbs where you get more freedom to play around with. On high-carb days, lessen your consumption of fats. On low-carb days, increase your consumption of fats. And make sure that you're doing all of that while still keeping your total daily caloric intake in mind. If you really want to lose weight on your designated schedule, then you need to stay strict with your daily caloric intake so that you are always able to hit the proper deficit numbers.

Step 7: Figure Out Your Menstrual Cycle Phases

Now, you need to start figuring out where you are on your menstrual cycle. Start plotting your phases. Again, the reason that this is essential for women to do is because your menstrual cycle can really impact the hormone levels of your body. And your capacity to burn fat and lose weight also largely depend on your hormone levels. So, in order for you to maximize your diet and your training, you have to be able to synchronize your health practices with your menstrual cycles appropriately.

Essentially, the first day of your menstrual cycle is the day of your first full blood flow. This cycle should last approximately 28 days. If you have an irregular period, you can always opt to just synchronize your diet with the lunar cycle as it also lasts for the same length of time.

Step 8: Plot Out Your High- and Low-Carb Days

This is a topic that has already been discussed exhaustively in a previous chapter. If you need a refresher on it, feel free to go back. However, for the short form, just remember that you are going to be primed to burn a lot of calories during the first two weeks of your cycle and then your body becomes more sluggish towards the final two weeks. So, you would want to situate more high- or moderate-carb days in the first two weeks. Then, you will want to incorporate more low-carb days in the final two weeks of your cycle.

Also, another general rule of thumb that you want to remember is that on your more active days, you have more liberty to consume carbohydrates. However, on recovery days or times when you don't really exert too much energy, it would be best for you to stick to low carb consumption so as to stay within a caloric deficit.

Step 9: Plan Your Meals Accordingly

At this point, you've already figured out a lot of things. By now, you know that there is some room for improvement with your body, and you have set goals for yourself moving forward. You know how many calories that you burn every day. You are now aware of what kind of caloric deficit you need to achieve and the numbers that you need to hit to achieve them. Because of your dedication to achieving your goals, you have decided that you want to form a workout routine and that you're sticking to it. You've also been oriented about how your menstrual cycles affect how your body processes calories and energy. So, you have developed a plan to sync your diet with your menstrual cycle, and you have all of the calculations planned out.

Now, it's just a matter of you putting real meals into the equation. Remember that all of your macros and your calories are mere numeric representations of the food that you eat. You have finally reached the step where you have to begin researching food and recipes that will help you form your meal plan for the week or even the whole month. If you are in need of some ideas for recipes, then you can refer to the following chapter of this book.

Step 10: Review Your Plan and Make Sure Everything Is Done Right

Lastly, you have to make sure that your plan is rock solid. Again, with carb cycling, half of the battle is done during the planning and preparation phases. If you get a few variables wrong in this initial phase, then you are potentially compromising your entire diet plan as a whole. It's very important that you go over your plan and check the numbers again. See if they all add up.

Also, along the way, feel free to revisit the plan and make a few tweaks here and there whenever you feel like it. A plan isn't designed to last forever. As you lose more weight, your body will undergo certain changes that could affect the variables that were involved in drafting your plan in the first place. With that, it's a good idea for you to revisit your plan every so often just to make sure that you are continuously optimizing your plan for weight loss and fat burn.

Best Food Sources for Carbohydrates

So, we've covered all of the basic reminders that you need to keep to heart while you're developing your plan. You've also been guided on the specific steps that you need to take to develop your carb cycling plan. You're practically set already. You've determined how many calories you need to be eating every day along with all of the macros that make up your calories. At this point, you should also already know when your high-carb and low-carb days should ideally be. Now, it's just a matter of you taking the time to do some research for recipes that you can use to fill up your eating schedule. Don't worry, this book has you covered on that front too. But more on the recipes later. Right now, you might just be thinking about what kind of food you will be eating on your high- and low-carb days.

Okay, there's one common misconception that people get whenever they get into carb cycling diets. You might think that on high-carb days, you have the freedom to drown yourself in bowl after bowl of ice cream. You might assume that it would be okay for you to have as much cake as you want during your high-carb days as long as you stay strict on your low-carb days. True enough, if you crunch the numbers correctly, you might be able to get away with losing weight even when you're eating cake and ice cream all of the time. However, that wouldn't be a holistic approach to overall fitness. Also, it's not sustainable.

There are just certain carb sources that you will want to avoid as much as possible, even during your high-carb days. It's important to stress that while you might be desperate to lose weight, getting leaner isn't always going to be the strongest indicator of overall health and wellness. So, for the purpose of still staying fit and healthy while carb cycling, here is a list of carbs that you need to eat and carbs you need to avoid while dieting.

Carbs to Eat

- bananas
- mangoes
- strawberries
- blueberries
- blackberries
- cherries
- lettuce
- cauliflower
- broccoli
- squash
- tomatoes
- papayas
- bitter gourds
- bean sprouts
- lemons
- avocados
- whole grains
- wheat pasta
- sweet potato
- whole wheat bread
- quinoa
- couscous
- amaranth, etc.

Carbs to Avoid

- white bread
- white rice
- ice cream
- fried potatoes
- refined sugar
- refined flour
- pastries
- cakes
- sugary sauces/dressings
- sodas
- sugary energy drinks
- alcoholic beverages, etc.

If we just keep on listing different kinds of food here, then the book will go on and on. But you get the general picture, right? As much as possible, when choosing your carb sources, try to keep it as fresh and as natural as possible. Go for foods that undergo little to no processing. Stay away from foods that are drenched in sugar or that have undergone substantial processing. Remember that weight loss isn't just a matter of keeping track of your calories. It's also about the quality of the food that you eat. If you eat better, your metabolic system just functions better, and you set yourself up for losing more weight in the future.

Again, take note that the ultimate goal here is health and wellness. Weight loss just plays a vital part of that, but it's not the priority. You can lose all the weight that you want, but if you're just munching on soda and ice cream throughout that period, you're not really healthy.

Final Thoughts

Be proud of yourself for taking that extra step. You've already come up with a rough plan for yourself to help you achieve all of your weight loss goals. Now, it's just a matter of polishing and fine-tuning your plan, and then actually executing it. That might be the scary part for a lot of people, but you shouldn't worry too much. The worst-case scenario is that you end up not achieving your weight loss goals, and you have to do the planning process all over again. That is a heck of a lot better than not even trying at all. However, if you really followed all of the lessons and principles that have been laid out in this book, it's unlikely that you're going to fail at this. Again, all of the tools and foundations are there. You just have to make sure that you are putting them all to good use.

But on the off chance that you do realize that the results just aren't what you're expecting, don't be afraid to go back to the drawing board to start over. There is no shame in going back to the start and finding out where you went wrong. It would be even more shameful if you just continue to stick to a plan that is obviously not working for you or if you just abandon dieting altogether.

Chapter 5:
High- and Low-Carb Recipes

Don't worry. You might already be freaking out if you're someone who isn't very confident about your culinary skills. The recipes that are listed in this book aren't all that complex or difficult. You won't need to undergo years of training in a culinary institute to be able to execute these meals properly. Also, these recipes are mere suggestions. You can always put your own spin on things and simplify them to your own personal preferences. However, these recipes are already pretty simple enough to begin with, so you don't have to worry too much about that.

In this chapter, various recipes will be given to cover the different meals of the day. One of the best aspects of carb cycling is that you don't really have to limit the amount of times that you eat in a day. It's merely a matter of controlling portion sizes. So, if you play your cards right, you can have three full meals plus a snack every day without worrying about getting fat or gaining weight. Also, aside from teaching you how to execute these meals in this kitchen, these recipes also come with serving size suggestions together with corresponding nutritional information. You will be given the values for macros and calories with these recipes so that you have a better idea of how you can insert these meals into your overall meal plan.

Again, don't be afraid of getting creative with these. After all, it's you who is going to be eating these meals in the end. Just know that any changes you make to the recipes might also result in changes of the numerical values of the nutritional info. With that said, here are some recipes for high- and low-carb meals that you can incorporate into your carb cycling plan.

Breakfast
4-Egg and Cheese Omelette with Toast Slices (Low Carb)

Servings: 1

Preparation Time: 5 minutes

Cook Time: 5 minutes

Ingredients:

- 1 tbsp olive oil
- 4 medium-sized eggs
- 1 ½ oz of cheese
- 2 slices of whole wheat bread
- salt and pepper to taste

Instructions:

1. Prepare a skillet and place it over medium heat and add olive oil.
2. Brush olive oil all around the skillet and allow to heat up.
3. While skillet is heating up, crack the four eggs into a large bowl and whisk thoroughly with a fork or eggbeater.
4. Then, add the eggs to the skillet and stir continuously as it cooks. Make sure to never stop stirring to prevent the eggs from becoming rubbery or tough.
5. Once the eggs are cooked, turn off the heat, and add the cheese to the eggs. Continue to stir to fully incorporate the cheese into the eggs.
6. Set the eggs on a plate and serve together with two slices of wheat bread.
7. Season the eggs with salt and pepper to taste.

Nutritional Information:

Calories: 383 kcal, Carbs: 36 g, Fat: 17 g, Protein: 21 g

Cream Cheese Pancakes (Low Carb)

Servings: 1

Preparation Time: 3 minutes

Cook Time: 9 minutes

Ingredients:

- 2 oz of cream cheese
- 2 eggs
- 1 tsp of low carb sweetener
- ½ tsp cinnamon powder

Instructions:

1. Prepare a high-power blender and add all of the ingredients.
2. Blend it all together on high until it achieves a smooth and thick consistency.
3. Allow to rest for 2 minutes so that the bubbles will settle.
4. Prepare a non-stick skillet and place it over medium heat.
5. Grease the pan with butter or non-stick spray.
6. Once the pan is hot, add ¼ of the batter to the pan in a clean circular shape.
7. Cook for two minutes or until it achieves a golden-brown color on the bottom.
8. Flip the pancake and allow the other side to cook for another minute.
9. Repeat this process until you run out of batter.
10. (Optional) Serve with low-carb syrup or berries as toppings.

Nutritional Information:

Calories: 344 kcal, Carbs: 3 g, Fat: 29 g, Protein: 17 g

Keto Coconut Porridge (Low Carb)

Servings: 1

Preparation Time: 5 minutes

Cook Time: 5 minutes

Ingredients:

- 1 large egg
- 1 tbsp of coconut flour
- 1 pinch of ground psyllium husk powder
- 1 oz butter (room temperature)
- 4 tbsp of coconut cream
- salt to taste

Instructions:

1. In a medium-sized bowl, add the egg and whisk until thoroughly beaten.
2. Then, add the coconut flour, psyllium husk powder, and salt to the mixture.
3. Prepare a small pan and place it over low heat. Melt the butter and coconut cream in the pan. Make sure that both ingredients are well incorporated.
4. Gradually add the egg mixture into the pan and mix thoroughly until you achieve a thick and creamy texture.
5. (Optional) Top your porridge with berries, nuts, or coconut shavings.

Nutritional Information:

Calories: 486 kcal, Carbs: 4 g, Fat: 49 g, Protein: 9 g

Fruity Oatmeal Bowl (High Carb)

Servings: 2

Preparation Time: 5 minutes

Cook Time: 5 minutes

Ingredients:

- 1 cup rolled oats
- natural sweeteners to taste (like honey)
- ¼ cup coconut milk
- 1 banana (sliced)
- ½ mango (peeled and thinly sliced)
- 1 kiwi (peeled and sliced)
- ¼ cup pineapple (diced)
- 2 tbsp raspberries
- 1 tbsp coconut flakes

Instructions:

1. Cook the oatmeal as directed on the package instructions.
2. Stir the coconut milk into the pot of oatmeal and add your desired amount of sweetener.
3. Incorporate the fruits into the oatmeal and garnish with coconut flakes.
4. Serve either chilled or warm.

Nutritional Information:

Calories: 348 kcal, Carbs: 59 g, Fat: 10 g, Protein:7 g

Lunch

Zucchini and Walnut Salad (Low Carb)

Servings: 4

Preparation Time: 5 minutes

Cook Time: 2 minutes

Ingredients:

For the Dressing:

- 2 tbsp olive oil
- ¾ cup mayonnaise
- 2 tsp lemon juice
- 1 clove of garlic (minced)
- ½ tsp salt
- ¼ tsp chili powder

For the Salad:

- 1 head of romaine lettuce
- 4 oz of arugula
- ¼ cup of chopped scallions
- 2 whole zucchinis
- 1 tbsp olive oil
- 3 ½ oz of chopped walnuts
- salt and pepper to taste

Instructions:

1. Prepare a small bowl and add all of the ingredients for the dressing.
2. Incorporate all of the dressing ingredients well and set aside.
3. In a large bowl, combine the trimmed romaine, arugula, and chives. Make sure that all of the ingredients are mixed well.

4. On a cutting board, split both zucchinis lengthwise and remove the seeds. Then, cut the zucchinis into small half-inch pieces crosswise.
5. Prepare a medium-sized skillet and place it over medium heat. Add olive oil to the pan and allow to heat until it shimmers. Then, add the zucchini pieces to the skillet and season with salt and pepper.
6. Allow the zucchini to cook until slightly browned on the outside. Then, add the nuts to the pan and cook both ingredients together.
7. Add the zucchini and the walnuts to the lettuce leaves and then drizzle with salad dressing.

Nutritional Information:

Calories: 595 kcal, Carbs: 8 g, Fat: 58 g, Protein: 9 g

Salad in a Jar (Low Carb)

Servings: 1

Preparation Time: 5 minutes

Cook Time: N/A

Ingredients:

- 1 oz of romaine lettuce
- ½ scallion
- 1 carrot
- 1 avocado
- 1 oz cherry tomatoes
- 1 oz red bell peppers
- 4 oz smoked salmon
- ¼ cup mayonnaise

Instructions:

1. Shred and chop all of the vegetables into reasonably small portions.
2. When assembling the salad in the jar, place the green and leafy vegetables at the bottom to serve as the base.
3. Add the other ingredients in their own respective layers.
4. Top the salad with the smoked salmon.
5. Add your dressing just before serving.

Nutritional Information:

Calories: 876 kcal, Carbs: 11 g, Fat: 76 g, Protein: 27 g

Moroccan Couscous with Flank Steak (High Carb)

Servings: 5

Preparation Time: 5 minutes

Cook Time: 10 minutes

Ingredients:

- 1 ¼ lb lean flank steak (chopped into 1-inch cubes)
- 1 tbsp olive oil
- 1 cup red onion (diced)
- 1 red bell pepper (diced)
- 1 ½ tbsp minced garlic
- ⅔ cup frozen peas
- ⅔ cup shredded carrots
- 1 ½ cup low-sodium beef broth
- 1 cup dry couscous
- 2 tbsp fresh mint
- ⅓ cup raisins
- 2 tsp smoked paprika
- 1 tsp cumin
- 1 tsp turmeric
- ½ tsp cayenne powder
- 1 tsp coriander
- ½ tsp cinnamon

Instructions:

1. Prepare a non-stick skillet and set it on high heat. Brush or spray the skillet with oil or non-stick spray and then add the beef cubes. Season the beef with salt and pepper. Allow the beef to sear on one side for one minute before shaking the pan to sear the other sides. Cook the beef until you've achieved your desired readiness and then remove it from the skillet.
2. Lower the heat to medium and add olive oil, garlic, salt, onions, bell pepper, and black pepper. Cook for around 2 minutes or until the onions become slightly translucent. Add all of the

powder spices to the pan and make sure that the onions and bell peppers are seasoned properly.

3. Add the frozen peas and carrots to the pan, and then immediately pour in the beef broth.
4. Bring the broth to a light simmer and add the couscous. Gently incorporate everything together inside of the broth and remove from the heat to allow the couscous to absorb the liquid. This should take no more than 5 minutes.
5. Mix in the beef and serve in equal portions.

Nutritional Information:

Calories: 371 kcal, Carbs: 41 g, Fat: 9 g, Protein: 32 g

Slow-Cooked Chicken and Rice Casserole (High Carb)

Servings: 5

Preparation Time: 10 minutes

Cook Time: 4 hours

Ingredients:

- 1 lb chicken breast (chopped into 1-inch pieces)
- 3 ½ cups low-sodium chicken broth
- 1 cup uncooked brown rice
- ½ cup 2% Greek yogurt
- ⅔ cup cheddar cheese
- 12 oz raw broccoli florets
- 1 tbsp olive oil
- 1 tbsp garlic (minced)
- ½ red onion (diced)
- 1 tsp thyme
- 1 tsp rosemary

Instructions:

1. Prepare a slow cooker and set it to a sauté function on low heat. Add the olive oil, onions, and garlic into the slow cooker until the onions are caramelized. This should take around 3 to 5 minutes.
2. Add the brown rice, thyme, and rosemary. Make sure that the spices are well incorporated into the brown rice.
3. Pour the chicken broth into the cooker and follow it with the raw chicken breasts. Cook the rice and chicken for around 3 to 5 hours.
4. When there's around 30 minutes to 1 hour left of cooking, stir the Greek yogurt and cheese into the slow cooker. Mix everything until the liquid becomes thick and creamy.
5. Place the raw broccoli on top of the rice, but do not mix it. Allow the heat to soften the broccoli.
6. Allow the entire meal to cook for the remaining time.

7. Season with salt and pepper and serve.

Nutritional Information:

Calories: 380 kcal, Carbs: 36 g, Fat: 11 g, Protein: 36 g

Dinner

Turkey Sandwich on Whole Wheat (Low Carb)

Servings: 1

Preparation Time: 20 minutes

Cook Time: N/A

Ingredients:

- 1 large lettuce head
- 2 slices of whole wheat bread
- 1 tsp of cream cheese
- ¼ red onion
- ¼ small cucumber (slices)
- 25 grams of sprouts
- 31 grams of sliced turkey ham (lean)
- salt and pepper to taste

Instructions:

1. Remove the lettuce leaves from the head and rinse thoroughly. Set the leaves aside and allow to dry.
2. While waiting for the leaves to dry, prepare the two slices of bread and spread the cream cheese evenly along the surface of one slice.
3. Take the cucumber and rinse thoroughly. Then, slice it into very thin portions.
4. Peel the onion and then rinse it thoroughly. Thinly slice the onion into rings.
5. Prepare the sprouts and rinse them thoroughly. Shake them to remove any excess water and allow to dry for a bit.
6. On a serving plate or cutting board, place the slice of bread without cream cheese on the bottom to serve as the base of the sandwich. Then, add the lettuce leaves and season with salt and

pepper. After that, proceed to add layers of ham, onions, cucumbers, and sprouts. Lightly season each layer along the way.

7. Top the sandwich with the remaining slice of bread and serve as is.

Nutritional Information:

Calories: 241 kcal, Carbs: 36 g, Fat: 4.5 g, Protein: 15.5 g

Fried Kale and Broccoli Salad (Low Carb)

Servings: 2

Preparation Time: 5 minutes

Cook Time: 10 to 12 minutes

Ingredients:

- ½ cup mayonnaise
- 1 tbsp whole-grain mustard
- 4 eggs
- ½ lb broccoli
- 4 oz of kale
- 2 scallions
- 2 garlic cloves
- 2 avocados
- 2 tbsp olive oil
- chili flakes, salt, and pepper to taste

Instructions:

1. Add water to a large pot and fill it up halfway. Submerge the unpeeled eggs into the pot of water and place the pot over medium heat. Bring the water to a light boil and allow the eggs to cook for 8 to 10 minutes.
2. While the eggs are cooking, prepare a large bowl of ice and water to serve as an ice bath for the eggs.
3. In a separate small bowl, mix the mayo and mustard together and set aside.
4. Once cooked, remove the eggs from the pot and place the eggs in the ice bath prior to peeling.
5. Once the eggs have cooled, peel them and slice them into halves or quarters.
6. Split the avocados in half. Remove the pits and cut the meat into slices.
7. Slice the cloves of garlic as thinly as you can and fry them up over a hot skillet with olive oil. Cook the garlic until they are

crispy and set aside on top of a paper towel.

8. Chop the kale and broccoli coarsely and cook in the frying pan together with butter. Fry the vegetables over medium-high heat until they have softened.

9. Add the kale and broccoli to a large bowl with avocados, eggs, and the mayo-mustard dressing. Season everything with salt, chili flakes, and pepper. Top it with crunchy garlic slices and serve.

Nutritional Information:

Calories: 1022 kcal, Carbs: 13 g, Fat: 94 g, Protein: 22 g

Sweet and Spicy Beef Bowl (High Carb)

Servings: 4

Preparation Time: 5 minutes

Cook Time: 15 minutes

Ingredients:

- 12 oz sugar snap peas
- 2 radicchio (chopped)
- juice from ½ lemon
- 2 cups of cooked brown rice
- 1 ½ lb flank steak (chopped into ½ inch cubes)

For the sauce:

- 3 tbsp low-sodium soy sauce
- 2 tbsp fresh ginger
- 2 tsp sesame oil
- 2 tbsp water
- 3 tbsp sriracha
- 4 tbsp coconut sugar
- juice from one whole orange
- 1 ½ tbsp arrowroot starch

For garnish:

- orange wedge
- sesame seeds
- chopped scallions

Instructions:

1. Mix together all of the ingredients for the sauce except for the arrowroot. Set the sauce and the arrowroot aside for the meantime.
2. Prepare a large non-stick pan and set it over high heat. Once the pan has heated, add the sugar peas first and cook until soft.

Make sure to continuously stir the peas so as to prevent charring on the outside. This should take around 3 minutes.

3. Remove the peas from the skillet once they are cooked. Then, add the radicchio to the pan. While the radicchio is cooking, add some lemon juice. Continue to cook until the radicchio begins to wilt. Once cooked, remove the radicchio from the pan.

4. Then, add the chopped beef into the pan and sear until it has achieved your desired readiness. Once the beef is cooked, reduce the heat of the pan and move the beef towards the sides, creating a big gap in the middle.

5. Add the arrowroot to your sauce and add the entire sauce mixture to the center of the skillet. Once the sauce begins to bubble or thicken, remove the pan from the heat and continuously fold the beef into the sauce.

6. Remove the beef from the pan and garnish with scallions and sesame seeds.

7. Add the beef on top of the brown rice and mix together with radicchio and sugar snap peas.

8. Divide into equal portions and serve.

Nutritional Information:

Calories: 459 kcal, Carbs: 45 g, Fat: 11 g, Protein: 40 g

Spicy Avocado Chicken Salad Wrap

Servings: 1

Preparation Time: 5 minutes

Cook Time: 5 minutes

Ingredients:

- 1 large whole wheat tortilla
- 4 oz cooked chicken breast (chopped)
- 1 ½ cups of chopped romaine lettuce
- ½ beefsteak tomato (chopped)
- ⅓ cup cucumber (chopped)
- ½ medium avocado (chopped)
- ¾ tbsp Cajun seasoning powder
- 2 tbsp plain yogurt

Instructions:

1. Place the chicken in a large bowl and season with the Cajun powder. Make sure that the chicken is well coated with the seasoning.
2. Add the rest of the ingredients into the bowl except for the tortilla.
3. Mix the contents of the bowl thoroughly with a spatula until they are all well incorporated.
4. Take the tortilla and warm it in the microwave for around 10 to 15 seconds. Take the tortilla out of the microwave and place it on a flat, stable surface.
5. Add the salad mix to the center of the tortilla and fold the sides together. Roll the entire tortilla until it forms a burrito.
6. Serve the burrito sliced or whole.

Nutritional Information:

Calories: 534 kcal, Carbs: 49 g, Fat: 18 g, Protein: 47 g

Snacks

Almond Milkshake (Low Carb)

Servings: 1

Preparation Time: 5 minutes

Cook Time: N/A

Ingredients:

- 1 oz of almonds
- 1 cup of full-cream milk
- 1 cup of ice cubes
- zero-calorie sweetener (Stevia, Splenda, etc.)

Instructions:

1. Add the ice cubes to a high-power blender and set it to crush.
2. Crush the ice until it achieves a snowy consistency.
3. Add the full-cream milk and the almonds to the blender and set it to blend.
4. Blend the ingredients until they are all well incorporated with one another.
5. (Optional) Add sweetener to the mixture and serve chilled.

Nutritional Information:

Calories: 264 kcal, Carbs: 20 g, Fat: 16 g, Protein: 14 g

Low-Carb Deviled Eggs (Low Carb)

Servings: 4

Preparation Time: 5 minutes

Cook Time: 12 minutes

Ingredients:

- 4 large eggs
- ¼ cup mayonnaise
- 1 tsp tabasco
- 8 strips of smoked salmon
- fresh dill and salt to taste

Instructions:

1. Add water to a large pot and fill it up halfway. Submerge the unpeeled eggs into the pot of water and place the pot over medium heat. Bring the water to a light boil and allow the eggs to cook for 8 to 10 minutes.
2. While the eggs are cooking, prepare a large bowl of ice and water to serve as an ice bath for the eggs.
3. Once cooked, remove the eggs from the pot and place the eggs in the ice bath prior to peeling.
4. Once the eggs have cooled, remove the shells and split the eggs in half. Scoop the yolk out of the eggs and place the yolks and whites on separate plates.
5. Mash the egg yolks with a masher or a fork and add salt, mayonnaise, and tabasco.
6. Once all of the ingredients in the egg yolk mixture are well incorporated, add them back to the egg whites and top with a small strip of smoked salmon.
7. Decorate each egg with dill and serve.

Nutritional Information:

Calories: 163 kcal, Carbs: 0.5 g, Fat: 15 g, Protein: 7 g

Peanut Butter Sandwich on Wheat Bread (High Carb)

Servings: 1

Preparation Time: 2 minutes

Cook Time: N/A

Ingredients:

- 2 tbsp of peanut butter
- 2 slices of whole wheat bread

Instructions:

1. Prepare the two slices of bread and arrange each slice on a stable surface.
2. Spread one tablespoon of peanut butter on each slice of bread.
3. Combine both slices together or eat them independently.
4. (Optional) Place the sandwich on top of a hot skillet and allow to cook for one minute on each side to make the bread crunchier.

Nutritional Information:

Calories: 327 kcal, Carbs: 30 g, Fat: 18 g, Protein: 15 g

Multigrain Bread with Olive Oil

Servings: 1

Preparation Time: 2 minutes

Cook Time: N/A

Ingredients:

- 1 tbsp olive oil
- 2 slices of multigrain bread
- salt to taste

Instructions:

1. Lightly toast multigrain bread in a toaster or on top of skillet.
2. Pour olive oil into a small dipping bowl and add salt to taste.
3. Break bread apart with hands and dip into olive oil prior to eating.

Nutritional Information:

Calories: 257 kcal, Carbs: 22.6 g, Fat: 16.2 g, Protein: 7 g

Chapter 6:
Tips and Tricks for Success

At this point, you should already have everything that you need to start your carb cycling diet plan. However, the book isn't over yet. We're not going to leave you hanging just yet. Just because you have everything that you need doesn't mean that you still won't stand to benefit from learning a few of the tips and tricks of the trade. Again, the road to success in weight loss and fitness isn't going to be without its fair share of bumps and hitches. You are bound to make a few mistakes here and there, but that's okay. That's a part of the process.

However, there are a few ways that you can minimize your chances of making mistakes. Here are a few tips and tricks that you can keep up your sleeve just to make sure that you are putting yourself in the best possible position to succeed.

Drink Lots of Water

For the very first tip, you need to make it a point to always hydrate. Water is life... quite literally. Did you know that water makes up 60% of your body? That fact alone should serve as enough incentive for you to up your water intake. When you drink lots of water, you are constantly hydrating your muscles and your vital organs. This means that your body is going to be able to function more efficiently for metabolizing food and for working out as well.

On top of that, water can also help curb hunger. A lot of the time, when people think that they're hungry, they're really just thirsty. So, the next time you think you're craving that fried chicken sandwich, reach for a glass of water instead. You will be surprised at how often you will be able to curb your cravings just by drinking a glass of water. Make sure that you always have a bottle or glass of water near you at all times. This way, it's much easier for you to always keep yourself hydrated.

Set Concrete and Realistic Goals

Goal setting is always going to be important in whatever endeavor you choose to engage in. Sure, when you're just starting out, it's so easy to set goals like *"I want to be healthier,"* or *"I want to lose a lot of weight,"* and that's fine. These are valid goals to have. However, when you're just starting out, it's important that you set goals that are more concrete and less ambiguous. Of course, you want to lose a lot of weight. But it would be better to attribute a specific number to that particular goal.

So, instead of saying that you want to lose an arbitrary amount of weight, put a real number to it. Say you want to lose 5 pounds next month. Say you want to lose 2 pounds this week. When you are shooting for concrete and realistic goals like this, it becomes a lot easier to track your progress. And it doesn't even just have to be about your weight. Here are a few examples of goals that you can set for yourself:

- I want to go five straight days without cheating on my diet.
- I want to be able to run 5 km in under 30 minutes.
- I want to fit back into my old pair of jeans.
- I want to wake up at 6 a.m. every day to work out.

When you have more specific and concrete goals like this, the whole process becomes a lot easier to absorb and digest.

Don't Pay Too Much Attention to the Scale

Okay, it's important to stress this point, especially since we've talked about setting more concrete goals for yourself. Yes, in the previous tip, you were advised to be more concrete about how much weight you want to lose. So, that means that you need to check your weight consistently to know if you're making progress. That's the right idea. However, too many people make the mistake of obsessing over the number that is on the scale. Keep in mind that weight loss is not a linear process. Your weight is going to keep on fluctuating. You will lose weight and you will gain it back. That's just the nature of weight loss.

So, if you keep on obsessing over the number that's on the scale, you might end up thinking that you're doing things wrong even though you're doing everything right. Instead of checking the scales every day, try doing so just once a week or every two weeks instead. Also, the scale only tells half the story. Remember that muscles are heavier than fats. So, if you're burning fat and you're gaining muscle, you might not be losing that much weight. But if that's the case, your body fat percentage is still going down and that's the ultimate goal. Also, another better indicator of true weight loss is checking your waistline. Sometimes, the number on the scale might not be going down so much. But if your waistline is getting smaller, that's a better indicator of more effective weight loss.

Do Meal Planning and Preparation

There's a reason why multiple chapters in this book have been dedicated to you really planning and preparing your meals in advance. Okay, there are two aspects of this tip. There is the planning aspect and there is the preparation aspect. Both aspects are equally important, and you really need to incorporate both habits into your life of health and wellness.

First, planning. With carb cycling, it's not just a matter of you deciding on the spot whether you will have a high- or low-carb day. You aren't going to find much success with this diet if you're going to go about it whimsically. You need to consciously plan your low- and high-carb days as you consider other factors of your lifestyle like training schedule, training intensity, and menstrual cycle. The old adage says that a failure to plan is a plan to fail. So, don't disregard the whole planning process of carb cycling.

Next, there is meal preparation. This tip is all about practicality. When you engage in meal planning, then you know all of the food that you're going to consume over an extended period. Since you already have that knowledge, it would also be best for you to prepare most of your meals in advance as well. This is going to save you the trouble of having to cook food up every single time you want to eat. Part of being able to stick to a diet is having healthy food readily available at any moment's notice. Most people find success in bulk cooking. They take one day out of every week, and they dedicate it to preparing ALL of the meals for that week. Of course, you can stagger your meals so that they're not always repetitive. It's all up to you.

Remember Fat Isn't the Enemy

Contrary to what many people believe, fat is actually not the enemy. Eating fat isn't going to make you fat. Again, this is a point that has already been proven time and time again by practitioners of the keto diet. Just because you're eating a lot of fat doesn't necessarily mean that that food is going to be processed into fat for your body. The real enemy here is sugar. Remember that sugar is what is converted into glucose and is used as energy for your body. However, if you eat too much sugar, a lot of that glucose doesn't get used up, and it gets converted into stored fat in the body.

Also, the thing about sugar is that it's so addictive and easy to consume. It can be so easy to go overboard on the calories from mere sugar consumption. This is why a diet plan like carb cycling, which directly manages and oversees the healthy consumption of carbohydrates and sugar, is so effective. Instead of vilifying fat, it would be better to demonize empty carbs like sugar instead.

Stick to a Solid Workout Plan

Training shouldn't be sporadic either. Again, with this kind of diet, it's really going to be at its most effective state if you pair it with a healthy training regimen. And when we say healthy training regimen, we're talking about an actual plan that you can stick to over a prolonged period. It's not enough that you decide to run a 5k today, rest a few days, and then join a yoga class when you feel like you have the energy. That's not what a workout plan is.

This is why goal setting is so important in fitness. For instance, if you make it a concrete goal for yourself to run a half-marathon in six months, then that means that you have to follow a strict running program for you to stay in shape. Maybe, if you make it a goal to attend five yoga classes per week, then that means you have a solid plan for yourself in terms of scheduling. Also, keep in mind that your low- and high-carb days are going to be dependent on what kind of workout plan you have. Again, this isn't just something that you can approach whimsically and expect to yield positive results.

Cook Your Own Meals

So, what is the best way for you to really know how much food you're eating? It's when you take the time to really measure and cook your own meals. Sure, you can always opt to go for the easier route by going to restaurants and ordering meals from there. However, what is easy isn't always going to be the most accurate. There's no way you can really gauge the macros and calories in a meal that you order from a restaurant because you weren't there during the cooking and preparation process.

Of course, there are also various healthy meal service providers out there who offer calorie-counted options for you. You can always opt to go that route as well. However, these services tend to be very pricey, and it might not be the practical thing for most people. This should only serve as the last resort when you don't think that you have the time or the skills to cook delicious, healthy meals for yourself. However, ultimately, anyone can cook to a certain degree. A lot of the recipes listed in this book are designed for beginners and novices in the kitchen. It's just a matter of taking the time to really master cooking these recipes.

Avoid Drinking Calories

Much to the dismay of many people, calories also exist in drinks. Yes. The one or two glasses of wine that you have after dinner are also going to bring calories with them as well. That bottle of Gatorade or Red Bull that you drank to fuel your workout? Those have calories in them as well. The thing about beverages like these is that they are incredibly deceptive. They pack a lot of calories, but they don't really do much good for the body from a nutrition standpoint. So, as much as possible just stick to water.

Of course, there are some beverages out there that have little to no calories at all like tea or coffee. Things only get dangerous when you start adding sweeteners or creamers to these beverages. If you must have a beverage other than water, you can always opt for tea or coffee. Also, the caffeine content of these beverages is known to help improve your metabolism and facilitate fat burn. Just make sure that you don't go overboard with adding artificial or natural sweeteners and creamers.

It would be much better if you get your calories from whole foods like lean proteins or whole grains.

Don't Go Grocery Shopping While Hungry or Without a Plan

This tip might seem rather silly, but there's actually real scientific backing to it. Whenever you are hungry, it's known that you don't really have the ability to think at your logical peak. This is because your mind is distracted, and it can't really focus on the tasks that it must accomplish. It's the same with grocery shopping too. You might think that it's such a menial task that it doesn't require much focus or logic. However, this is where you would be wrong.

If you go into a grocery store while you're hungry, your mind will trick itself into thinking that you should be buying things that you don't really need. Ideally, you will go into a grocery store with a set grocery list and just stick to that. You won't choose things on a whim. You might end up buying a lot of unnecessary or unhealthy food items that could potentially compromise your diet. So, the best course of action will be for you to fill yourself up before visiting the grocery store. And make sure that you have a grocery list ready. Stick to that list!

Evolve Your Goals Along the Way

Earlier in this list, you were taught that you need to really be serious about setting your goals before you embark on your fitness journey. However, please know that your goals are never set in stone and that they are subject to occasional changes and evolution. Again, as you become fitter and leaner, your body is going to undergo some very significant changes. These changes are all for the better, of course. However, that also means that a lot of the goals that you set at the start might become obsolete. This is why it's essential that you continuously evolve your goals along the way.

For instance, if you had your sights set on losing 10 pounds in one month originally, perhaps you can taper it down to 7 or 8 pounds in the next month. Your body is going to find it difficult to burn more fat the leaner it gets. So, it would be smart for you to taper your weight loss goals gradually as you go. Another example is if you make it a goal to run a half-marathon. Naturally, if you complete that goal, then you might want to evolve and aim for running a full marathon. If you constantly evolve your goals, then you will realize the work is never done. In this sense, you keep pushing for self-improvement and development.

Don't Give Up on a Diet Too Quickly

This is a common mistake that a lot of people make whenever they're just starting out. Keep in mind that everyone's body is going to function differently. This means that not all people are going to yield the same results or responses towards a certain diet. Just because you have a friend who lost weight in two weeks from carb cycling doesn't mean that it's going to be the same for you. Sometimes, the effects take much longer for other people. There are a variety of factors to consider here such as genetics, lifestyle, and hormones. Ultimately, you will only really be able to see the effects of a diet after at least three to four weeks of strict dieting. If you cheat along the way, then the results might be delayed even further.

Just stick to it. Make sure that you are staying strict with your diet for at least three to four weeks. Don't have any cheat days and see if there are results. If it doesn't work for you, then maybe the plan was off to begin with. Try to make a few adjustments and lower the caloric values for your consumption a bit. If it still doesn't work, then maybe it just isn't a good fit. And that's okay. There's no shame in that. It will only be a waste if you abandon the diet too quickly without ever giving it a chance.

Find Yourself a Diet or Training Buddy

Like love, fitness is something that is best when shared. Of course, you are perfectly capable of achieving all of your goals and dreams on your own. You don't have to be reliant on anyone else to help you achieve your fitness goals. No one is going to do the work for you, and so, no one should ever get to tell you that you can't do something. However, it always helps whenever you have a strong support system. So, if you can recruit a few friends or buddies to help keep you accountable to your goals and duties, then that's good.

Again, it's important to emphasize that you can do everything on your own. But if you have an opportunity to gain the help and support of other people, that is always a plus. You can keep each other honest, and you can celebrate each other's victories. Also, there is this understated energy that you can get from knowing that other people are invested in your success as well. It's a lot more comforting to face a tough journey knowing that you have other people at your side who are willing to help you out.

Stick to Workouts or Diets You Really Enjoy

If you don't have fun doing it, then it's not worth doing. Of course, if you had the choice, in an ideal world, you would be able to eat anything that you want without having to worry about getting fat. Unfortunately, this is not the world that we live in. So, you have to abide by certain fitness rules and principles if you want to remain healthy. However, just because you need to abide by these rules doesn't mean that you won't get the opportunity to have fun in the process. It's important that in your health and fitness journey, you still enjoy what you're doing.

When you're choosing a workout program, it should be physically strenuous enough so you're achieving results. However, it should also be an enjoyable experience for you so that it becomes more sustainable. When selecting a diet program, it has to be strict in the sense that you are adhering to proper nutritional principles. However, it shouldn't be a diet that makes you sad and depressed about life. You should still have a pretty positive and healthy relationship with your food. This is why a flexible diet like carb cycling just works so well for a lot of people. It's not as restrictive as other diets, but it still instills a sense of discipline.

Schedule Your Cheat Days

Okay, this might seem like it's counterintuitive, but there is some logic behind this. As much as possible, you won't want to have any cheat days ever. If it's possible for you to stay strict on your diet forever, then that's a good thing. However, to be quite frank about it, a vast majority of people don't have that kind of willpower. Occasionally, we are going to be entitled to a cheat day and that's okay. Life is meant to be enjoyed, after all. It's all just a matter of keeping things in moderation.

Having said that, it is better if you actually schedule your cheat days instead of just deciding on the spot that you're going to cheat. For example, some people find it effective to stay very strict from Monday to Saturday and then have their cheat days on Sunday. Other people would find it more effective to have one cheat day every two weeks or even just once every month. It all depends. Just make sure that your cheat days aren't getting in the way of your progress. If you have this kind of system in place, you are more motivated to stay strict on the days that you're supposed to be strict.

Get Better Sleep at Night

Lastly, it's very important that you get proper sleep at night. Your sleeping patterns can dramatically impact the way that your body functions. You might not know this, but having poor sleeping patterns can actually impair your metabolic system and result in you retaining more weight. Lacking sleep can result in lower insulin sensitivity, and so your body starts to retain more fat instead of burning more of it. Also, in addition to that, when you lack sleep, you just lack that energy to go work out and be active. Sleep is vital to a body's recovery and rejuvenation. When you don't get to sleep properly at night, your body doesn't get the chance to recuperate the way that it's supposed to. And this can negatively affect athletic performance.

Final Thoughts

Of course, these are only a few tips and tricks that you can use on your own fitness journey. You can choose whether or not to adopt them in your own life. You may also opt to develop your own systems. The only thing that matters here is that you find something that works best for you. It's ultimately about what you can yield from your own personal journey.

A lot of people don't realize that their fitness journeys are also deeply personal ones. A lot of your success is dependent on the kind of relationship that you have with your body, training regimen, and food. And like in real life relationships, there are some relationships that are healthy and there are others that are toxic. Make sure that all of your relationships are wholesome and positive. This way, you always know that you are feeding more positivity into your life and your daily habits.

Author's Note

We're nearing the end of this book, and it's been such an amazing journey. Hopefully, you will have come to learn a lot of things about the way that your body works and what you can do to make the most out of the body that you've been given. If you feel like you have had a great experience with reading this book, please do take the time to leave a short review on Amazon.

Reviews are really not easy to come by. And as an independent author who is working on a small budget, I have to rely on people like you to leave short and honest reviews of my work on any book-selling platform (Amazon, for example). These reviews serve as the lifeline for my career. I genuinely still want to be of help to many people out there and I need your reviews to keep me afloat. It could even just be a simple sentence or two. I don't want it to be too much of a bother for you.

With that said, I am grateful for you taking the time to read this book in its entirety. It's very heartwarming to know that you were patient enough to heed my advice on this matter. All the best to you and I wish you well on your road to fitness!

Conclusion

There you have it. Those are all of the essentials of learning about carb cycling for women. First of all, congratulations to you for deciding that you still have room for learning and development when it comes to health and wellness. That is always going to be an important first step. It's always essential that people realize that they don't know everything when it comes to their bodies. It takes great humility to pick up a book like this and acknowledge that there is so much left to learn about the ways that our bodies work.

Yes, it's true that the state of obesity in the world can be very saddening and alarming. There are so many people who have been gravely affected by obesity and all its mistresses. People have found the quality of their own lives severely compromised because of their poor eating habits and unhealthy lifestyles. Loads of individuals all over the world have lost their loved ones as a result of diseases or illnesses brought about by obesity. It really is one of the world's greatest killers, and we all need to fight back against it.

Of course, this book isn't saying that carb cycling is *the way* to go for *everyone* in the world. Again, we all find success in many different paths and methodologies. There is no one ideal diet that is best for everyone to follow. There are certain strengths and caveats to each of them. The only proper answer to what the best diet in the world is, is the one that works best for you. It's that simple. So, if you are someone who has managed to find a large degree of success through carb cycling, then that's good. Try to stick with it and be consistent. However, if it doesn't work for you, then that's okay too. The point here is that you are trying and that you're making an effort to improve your own personal health. By doing so, you are also uplifting the state of health and wellness all over the world in your own little way.

Getting fit and healthy isn't the easiest thing to do. Heck, if it were so easy, then everyone in the world would be fit and healthy, right? This is why it's even more important for people like you to really be more conscious about the little habits and routines that you incorporate into your daily life. Earlier in this book, it was mentioned that in order for you to find success, you need to live a life that is more purposeful and structured. That's really the truth, especially when it comes to health and wellness. If you do something that doesn't really add value or serve a purpose to your life, then you are just wasting energy. If you are putting forth unstructured efforts that are inconsistent, then you are wasting energy. One of the greatest keys to being consistent with your success in your health and fitness journey is adding a sense of structure and purpose.

Through it all, there will be various books, articles, journals, and other forms of media out there telling you that their recommended path for fitness is better and more effective. That might actually be true for some people. And it might even be true for you. Never be afraid of learning. Always be willing to open yourself up to opportunities for growth and development, especially in your fitness. If you have an opportunity to learn about a better practice for your health and wellness, then you should capitalize on it.

At the end of the day, it should be your responsibility to yourself to always try to keep up to date on the current and relevant information surrounding physical fitness. It would be an awful waste if you just completely disregard your body and take it for granted. As the old cliché goes, your body is a temple. You should always do your part in making sure that it is cared for.

Even if you have all sorts of problems going on in your life, you can always control how you treat your body. This is a truth that is consistent with everyone. You might be faced with a lot of uncontrollable circumstances, but you can always control how your body chooses to respond to those circumstances. Truthfully, if you take the time to consciously be healthier and fitter, you will find that everything in life just becomes a lot easier. You get a lot more energy and you feel more motivated to do more things. There's a reason why they say that exercise is a natural drug. The rush of endorphins will give you the natural high that you need to really enjoy the life that you've been given.

So, don't throw away your opportunity at living your best life. Regardless if it's with carb cycling or not, just make an effort to be fitter and healthier. You will only thank yourself in the long run for doing so. Fight to be a healthier you. Fight to live in a fitter society. Fight to be a part of a healthier world.

References

Collova, A. (2019, November 2). *IIFYM (If it fits your macros).* https://www.iifym.com/iifym-calculator/iifym-carb-cycling/

GBD 2017 Diet Collaborators. (2019, April 3). Health effects of dietary risks in 195 countries, 1990–2017: a systematic analysis for the Global Burden of Disease Study 2017. Retrieved from https://secure.jbs.elsevierhealth.com/action/cookieAbsent?code=null #%20

Family Health Team. (2019, August 13). *What to eat if you're carb cycling.* https://health.clevelandclinic.org/what-to-eat-if-youre-carb-cycling/

Health to Empower. (2015, August 13). *Carb cycling and weight loss for women.* https://www.healthtoempower.com/carb-cycling-and-weight-loss-for-women/

Hunter, G. T. (2018, August 14). *Carb cycling can boost workouts and weight loss (but there's a catch).* https://www.getthegloss.com/article/the-pros-and-cons-of-carb-cycling-for-better-workouts-and-weight-loss

Kallmyer, T. (2019, September 27). *How to calculate your macros to transform your body.* https://healthyeater.com/how-to-calculate-your-macros

Krupp, A. (2020, February 24). *Cycle syncing: Matching your health style to your menstrual cycle.* https://www.healthline.com/health/womens-health/guide-to-cycle-syncing-how-to-start#four-phases-of-cycle-syncing

Mawer, R. M. (2017, June 12). *What is carb cycling and how does it work?* https://www.healthline.com/nutrition/carb-cycling-101#section1

Natural Fit Foodie. (2019, November 8). *How to cycle sync your diet (with recipes)*. https://naturalfitfoodie.com/eat-menstrual-cycle/

Ryan, D., Candeias, V., & Jorgensen, L. (2018, May 17). *We need to change the way we think about obesity.* https://www.weforum.org/agenda/2018/05/we-need-to-change-the-narrative-around-obesity-heres-why/

Sweet, J. (2018, August 3). *What is carb cycling and does it work? Here's what experts say.* https://www.healthyway.com/content/what-is-carb-cycling/

CPSIA information can be obtained
at www.ICGtesting.com
Printed in the USA
LVHW011040080920
665299LV00016B/260

9 781734 697537